PRAISE FOR *A GUIDE*
TO CONSCIOUS MENOPAUSE

GW00645301

"This generous book is packed with practices, self-care and help for symptoms: a giant permission slip to love yourself through menopause transition in your way and your own timing."

Kate Codrington, author of *Second Spring*

"If you are hoping to navigate your way through a conscious menopause transition this book is going to be such a sturdy ally. It will encourage you to turn within, with the assurance of a gentle hand on your back as you find your way forward. Reva really understands what is asked of us during this great initiation, sharing wise insight, practical tips and guiding us to contemplations to help us find our own way through. My wish is for all midlife menopausal mavens to find this real, grounded, gem of a guide, to assist us through this powerful transition to wise woman. It is gold."

Susanna Guest, menstruality & menopause mentor,
co-author of *Wild Wisdom Journal*

"A wonderful book to empower and support women through the rite of passage that is menopause. Sharing her wealth of knowledge and experience, Reva challenges cultural stereotypes and shows how the menopause is a powerful initiation providing an opportunity to step into our authentic selves. Packed with practical advice and potent self-care practices, this is a superb book to help women move forward gracefully into their wise woman phase."

Carole Guyett, herbalist, medicine woman, and author of *Sacred Plant Initiations* and *The Herbalist's Guide to Pregnancy, Childbirth and Beyond*

"This book touches on a variety of approaches and tools addressing multiple aspects of menopause. A great tool for preparing and navigating what can be a beautiful transition in life. Taking up a new attitude and practices to support you can then be shared with younger women bringing more harmony and gentleness into life. Enjoy!"

Myra Lewin, founder and director of Hale Pule Ayurveda and Yoga, author of *Freedom in your Relationship with Food*

A GUIDE TO CONSCIOUS MENOPAUSE

A GUIDE TO CONSCIOUS MENOPAUSE

Passage to Wise Woman

Revā Adie

AEON

First published in 2023 by
Aeon Books

Copyright © 2023 by Revā Adie

British Library Cataloguing in Publication Data

A C.I.P. for this book is available from the British Library

ISBN-13: 978-1-80152-068-3

Typeset by Medlar Publishing Solutions Pvt Ltd, India

www.aeonbooks.co.uk

To all the women who have walked before me
and to those who will walk after me

Golden Thread
By Revā

My womb is made of golden thread,
golden thread, golden thread.

I sing my song of dreams met,
dreams met, dreams met.

I dance my dance of secrets kept,
secrets kept, secrets kept.

I spin my yarn of love's embrace,
love's embrace, love's embrace.

I weave my thread from birth to death,
birth to death, birth to death.

My womb is made of golden thread,
golden thread, golden thread.

CONTENTS

INDEX OF DIAGRAMS AND ILLUSTRATIONS

INTRODUCTION

The menopause is a unique journey. I would like to preface this guide by saying I'm not an expert. Like all of us I am an ordinary, and extraordinary, woman doing her best to navigate this human life and the menopause. This book has been birthed primarily from my own experience and also from what has been gathered over many years of listening to other women sharing their experiences. This book offers you some of the teachings that I have gratefully received as a psychotherapist, yoga teacher, ayurvedic advisor, and shamanic practitioner. It is drawn from my own journey and all the beautiful, varied strands of experience that I have received. Hopefully it is written in a way that if you are unfamiliar with these traditions, you will be able to follow, it is not necessary to have experience in these paths. Although yoga and shamanism may initially seem divergent paths, I have found them to be extremely complimentary and helpful to utilise both on my journey.

I have always been drawn to the esoteric end of traditions, including having more understanding about how energy moves and how this understanding can support us as energetic beings in physical form. Like many, I believe that everything is energy, and that energy has a vibration. Some is denser than others and this creates form and matter.

From this perspective everything is fluid and has the capacity to change, this includes our health, experiences, and our reality.

The foundation I have had as a psychotherapist has meant I have been privileged to hold space for many women individually, in groups and on retreats. In these sharings, women have had the courage to speak their truth and share authentically about the different phases of their lives including the menopause and the changes and experiences it has given them.

I incorporate anecdotes from my own journey, including a year living off grid in the Pembrokeshire woods. I chose to take this time to retreat primarily to have a *conscious menopause* and I was fortunate to have the freedom from responsibilities to do this. In the year before this, I felt an increasing need to be in nature, to follow my own routine and energy throughout my day rather than fit into an externally given or expected routine. Eventually, the call became so loud I had no choice. It was a childhood dream come true, a straw bale hut deep in the ancient woodland, surrounded by wild and unspoiled nature. There was a stream in front of the hut where I collected water and bathed. There is such beauty in simplifying. However, it is also easy to romanticise about such experiences, the romance and beauty is true but there are also challenges, some of which I have described in the book as illustrations of my own menopause process. I had hoped I would be guided by a wise woman but what I found was that I was confronted by self-sufficiency, my core wounds and the call to deepen my relationship with my inner being or teacher. I have included paintings that I created whilst in the wood to illustrate the guide. These were made at the time for my own use, a pictorial diary.

This book offers alternative perspectives on how to view and perceive the menopause from those which we are commonly given in mainstream society. It is a holistic smorgasbord, primarily because that is what I have found useful in my own personal journey. The book is an endeavour to support you in your conscious menopause, to challenge the prevailing perceptions and attitudes, the social conditioning that we have ingested from our mothers and grandmothers, our communities, teachers, leaders and media. We have inherited many thoughts, beliefs, and attitudes about the menopause and the majority have not been helpful in terms of us navigating these often-turbulent waters.

When I refer to a conscious menopause, I use the term to mean that you have your eyes wide open. You want to understand your experiences as fully as possible, with your whole self. You have gathered the available information, tuned into your own wisdom and knowing of what you need and then navigated it as skillfully, authentically and with as much heart as possible. For some of you, you may have already remembered how to listen to your own guidance, for others I hope that this book will support you in relaxing and opening into this.

During menopause a common feeling is that you're losing it, that you are going mad. You may find yourself asking yourself, 'am I going crazy or is this a spiritual initiation?' Since moving into my own peri-menopause, I have suspected that menopausal women would have been put into asylums and labelled insane in days gone past. Can you imagine how it must have been so socially perturbing and unaccept-able in the early 19th century to have a Lady raging, or refusing to get out of bed, or crying for seemingly no reason. I was pleased to see that Rosalyn Jones was exploring the same thread.

> "Women were expected to be quiet and polite and not disagree with the men in their lives—fathers and husbands. They were seen as hysterical and in need of treatment if they should dare to speak out or argue." (Jones, 2022)

The term 'hysteria' was used broadly to encompass all states shown by women that did not comply with the roles and expectations consigned by the patriarchy.

> "Historically, women would have been given a full hysterectomy or put in an asylum in the hope that they would return to 'normal ...'" (Jones, 2022)

The threat of being ostracised and incarcerated may explain why many women have not felt able to openly explore and express their meno-pausal experience. I recall hearing that my paternal Grandmother had been given electroconvulsive therapy. I was unable to get any further details other than a broad notion that she had been depressed. I was left wondering, was this diagnosed and prescribed during her menopause? How much had she been involved in this decision? Perhaps you have similar stories in your family.

From a mainstream perspective, when we think of the crone or wise woman, we conjure up images of an 'old hag' and scary 'witch' with negative connotations. Such archetypes are found cross-culturally.

They are universal symbols that are so embedded into our culture through stories, myth, literature, and art that they appear in our dreams and become rooted in our psyche. It is no wonder then that to begin to change our perceptions about the menopause is a huge process.

In recent years, there has been increased awareness about the menopause and its process and impact on women; this has been most welcome. However, the overriding message is still one of symptom management and relief, usually through medication, such as hormone replacement therapy (HRT). The focus being to allow women to continue to function at work and within their families with as little disruption as possible. Although this may be sought by many women, the irony is that the soul may be calling for disruption, that a smoothing over or dampening down of the wild woman can activate more distress, which if unheeded can lead to disease and disharmony in bodies, mind, and environment.

I sometimes refer to the menopause as 'beyond the thrust' because it describes where you get to as a menopausal woman, both in terms of engagement with life and sexuality. In your thirties and perhaps forties, you are generally content to move along with the thrust of life, the energy of this society as being one focused on achievement, action, delivering, and being on the ball. Of course, there may be times when you know inside that it's a ridiculous charade and you'd rather not play along, but you do so because everyone else is. But during the menopause that falls away and no longer works. With the changes to our physical and internal landscape we are forced to search for new purpose and meaning. With a change in hormones our sexual energy, desires, and choices may also change, which can have a profound impact on ourselves and our relationships. This is explored in Chapter 6, 'The Priestess Steps Up'.

This book offers a response to the call of many women to listen deeply to this passage and to the wisdom of their bodies. An acknowledgement and reorientation to this life phase as a *rite of passage*. Pivotal changes in our lives including birth, puberty, marriage, childbirth, and death are cross-culturally recognised as significant for the individual and community as a whole. Generally, society offers support, which often includes a ritual, ceremony, and celebration. This usually involves asking God, Source, or Spirit to support this profound passage. However, this is not the case with menopause—there has been a denial and a distortion which has meant that many women have felt unsupported and disconnected from their community or tribe.

These key life transitions can be a profound process in the human journey and in your own evolution, bringing both challenges and gifts. The experience of childbirth can be painful, the experience of pregnancy demanding and yet women do not shy away from it or avoid it (unless they make a conscious decision to do so or are unable to conceive) because there is a knowing that the gifts from this rite of passage, the exhilaration, expansion, and learning is both wanted, amazing, and needed. Similarly, the passage of menopause can be perceived as a necessary and welcome change.

When you ask many women what their menopause was like often, they say, 'I don't remember'—it's like a silent agreement that has been passed down through the generations. Then, with a little searching, they can recall night sweats, anxiety at work, and then taking hormone replacement therapy. It is rare to meet a role model and I am hoping that this book will support women to become the role model for the next generation. For most of us, we have not known women who have walked before us and who can share how they traversed this stage of life consciously and skillfully. This is partly why it can feel positive to navigate as best as we can, knowing that we will be able to share with our daughters, nieces, and sisters to support them in ways that we may not have been supported. This is part of *the change*, the stepping up as teacher, guide, and wise woman, knowing that even with our imperfections that we can offer our experience and unique wisdom when called for.

At the end of each chapter there are several contemplation questions as a prompt to support you in reflection and going deeper into your own process. They are starting points to your personal exploration that will probably lead to other contemplations and questions. If you have a friend or circle of women who you are resonating with, it can be satisfying to discuss these themes together, being a witness for one another. You may also find it helpful to write your reflections in a journal or create images in response to your contemplations and insights.

In every chapter there are also suggested practices to support a deepening of your exploration of your experience. Although these practices are linked with a specific phase of menopause and chapter content, they can be used at any time that feels right for you. You may wish to join them together to make a longer practice or do certain ones at certain times depending on how you are feeling. Some of the longer practices, such as the meditations and yoga nidras, are available as a guided audio recording at School of the Sacred Feminine website (see Further Resources on page 171). Some of the practices use visualisation, but do not worry if you consider yourself not to be a visual person, it may be that you sense things. Also, be open to changing your perception, we all use our imagination; as someone once told me, we can easily imagine what we want to eat for supper! With all the practices the ultimate and primary practice is to listen to yourself, to follow your own energy, and care for yourself. That means avoiding pushing, comparing, and criticising yourself as much as possible.

Much of the content has been gleaned from the wonderful and courageous sharing from women whom I have had the privilege to hold space for, both as a psychotherapist, retreat and course leader. I recall and apologise to some of the menopausal women in my early group psychotherapy days, as I did not always understand and recognise the significance and nature of the transition that they were in. This is an excellent reminder that a twenty- or thirty-year-old is unlikely to resonate and comprehend the complexity of the menopausal journey. One of the peculiar things that can happen, like a divine joke, is that a teenager's adolescence and menarche, the initiation marked by the onset of menstruation, can happen at the same time as her mother's menopause initiation. These are both times that need to be self-orientated and need self-care, retreat, and deep understanding. Both phases can have plenty of fire, insights, anxiety, and fears. From this perspective, it is easy to see how collisions are commonplace.

Another life event that is common during menopause is the aging, illness, and death of a parent or parents. My own father died during my menopause, and this reinforced a feeling of my foundations being shaken, of not being held by the masculine, feeling vulnerable and disconcerted. This can also mean that women may have to become careers at the very time when they need to release and relinquish their responsibilities.

Throughout the process it is helpful to maintain a sense of trust and wider perspective. At times this will be difficult to hold but knowing that all things pass and change can be reassuring and comforting.

Some of the book you will resonate with and other parts you may not do so. This sharing is an invitation to take what is supportive to you and leave to one side what isn't, and this may vary at different times through your menopause journey. Although the book is laid out to reflect the general sequence of menopause your experience may be different, so read different chapters and practices as and when you are called.

Which Witch Wytch Word

Finding the right language and words to express our experiences can be difficult and some terms can have various meanings—here are a few clarifications.

At times, I will refer to the feminine energy as *Shakti* and the masculine energy as *Shiva*. These terms are from the yogic and tantra traditions. Shiva in most yoga traditions is regarded as pure consciousness, as pure witness. Shakti is everything that exists and She permeates all that exists. In some Shakti traditions, such as the Kaula path, both Shakti and Shiva are perceived as pure consciousness and Shakti gives form to Shiva. This later perspective resonates with me as it aligns with the notion that the underlying principle is the Great Mother, the feminine principle. Of course, ultimately, even this division is transcended and there is no separation between Shakti and Shiva.

The book is written from a cis-het[1] perspective, as that is where the majority of my experience lies. The practices in the book can be adapted for same sex or non-binary individuals. At times I will refer to the feminine or masculine essence or qualities. These refer to the two energies that we all have whether born into a female or male body. Usually, we identify as being more aligned with either the feminine or masculine essence. We experience balance when we can integrate both of these energies.

Women's genitals have been vilified and shamed for many centuries. We may wish to reflect upon societies language and feel into what language feels honouring for us. The word *cunt* has become a swear word with negative connotations and many women choose to reclaim the word from its derogatory distortion. Vagina feels too medical, so for me and for the purposes of this book *yoni* seems the most appropriate word for woman's genitals. The term yoni can refer to the vagina and, or the womb. Similarly, to find the right language for the male genitals is also tricky—*cock, prick, penis* or *lingam* all have a different energy. I have chosen the words yoni and lingam as they seem to encompass both the physical nature of the genitalia, whilst also honouring them as sacred and energetic.

---

[1] A person that identifies as the gender they were assigned at birth and is romantically and sexually attracted to people of the opposite sex who are usually also cis-gendered or cis-sexual.

When I refer to the womb I do so not as a physical area but as an energetic space. This is still relevant to you even if you have had a hysterectomy. I am referring to the womb space and its gifts as a creative, fertile, wise vessel or cauldron.

I also want to differentiate my use of the term *conscious* and *Consciousness*. I use the spiritual term Consciousness to refer to the pure, universal, supreme non-duality, the space in which we and everything arises, dissolves, and returns. This is different from the use of the word conscious to describe the psyche or internal landscape of the mind, as in having awareness of, and the *unconscious*, which refers to that which is hidden and unknown.

Cosmic cycles

The Celtic festivals offer us a structure to orientate around and they also feed our connection with nature and her rhythm. The quarter festivals are the Spring and Autumn Equinox and the Summer and Winter Solstice. In between these are the cross-quarter festivals: Imbolc, Beltane, Lammas, and Samhain. Each one having a different quality and focus in relation to the natural cycle. The Earth's Cycle of Celebration by Glennie Kindred (Kindred, 1991) is a nice introduction. As we reconnect to these traditional celebrations, we are tapping into an ancient vein that supports us in the flow of life.

The moon relates to the feminine essence and emotional world. She waxes and wanes during the course of a month and this cycle has been a useful rhythm for us to follow for thousands of years. Increasingly, more women are following their menstrual cycle with awareness and using the moon and the seasons to skillfully navigate their own cycle. At times in this guide, I refer to the moon bleed map, relating our menstrual experiences to the natural rhythms of nature. These are general reference points and always from the understanding that every woman is unique. Although it can be helpful to share and discuss experiences and symptoms, making comparisons with others can encourage a feeling that you, or your body's intelligence has got it wrong. However, this is not the case—we are all unique and there are a range of cycles between women.

As we move into our menopause journey, we begin to adjust how we relate to the moon and seasonal cycle as our own menstrual cycle shifts. Just as our menstrual cycle is unique, so too is our menopause journey.

Some women like to refer to the menopause as their *moonpause*. As mentioned previously, finding the language that resonates can be difficult and highlights how language continues to be rooted in the masculine. Finding the language that feels good enough for you can be important. Profound transition points in our lives transcend rights, wrongs, and shoulds and part of the process is to continuously loosen and free ourselves from such concepts.

In astrological terms, we are moving from the Age of Pisces into the Age of Aquarius. The age of Aquarius brings a new world and paradigm. Many believe that this is a time of expanded consciousness and where the Divine Feminine is reclaiming Her power. This is perhaps reflected in the increased awareness of the menstrual cycle and menopause experience. Arguably, we are at a time where many of us are becoming more aligned to a higher vibration. Some astrologers, philosophers, and spiritual teachers believe that there is an invitation at this time of transition for us to step into our sovereignty. At times there will be reference to astrology, particularly in Chapter 5, 'Chiron is in the House' when we discuss the Chiron Return. Astrology can offer a helpful context to perceive your experience from.

Yoga and tantra

Yoga developed out of tantra, and tantra has much in common with shamanism. Often in the West we inaccurately associate tantra with permissive sexuality and yet tantra is vast and subtle, encompassing honouring of the feminine principle and acceptance of our wholeness, including the range of different mind states and sensory experiences. Yoga and tantra, as in many other traditions honour the forms of the Goddess. These are invoked through meditation, chanting, mantra, and prayer. The Goddesses are expressions of Shakti and are revealed in many guises. We are all expressions of Shakti, and the Goddess can support us in exploring different aspects, developing love, devotion, and worthiness for ourselves. There are many faces and names for the Goddess. In this book I refer to four Goddesses as they are the four who I know most and feel that they embrace the primary aspects of our personality and journey. Sally Kempton's *Awakening Shakti* is excellent to explore our relationship to these deities in more depth.

During my menopause, I found invoking Goddess Kali useful, particularly when in the eye of my menopause. I deeply related to Her, she said it was ok, that everything was falling away, being incinerated, she reminded me that death did not need to be avoided but could be embraced. To change I had to go through purification and the *fire of yoga*. In yoga, this is referred to as *tapasya*—the generation of heat and energy traditionally through disciplined practice and austerities. However, this fire of spiritual transformation can be considered to occur naturally and spontaneously as we navigate our spiritual journey. Goddess Kali and her capacity to support us through this fire is explored further in Chapter 3, 'The Underworld'. Similarly, Goddess Durga supported me to find the courage deep inside to keep taking a step forward, to trust that I was in a process where there would be victory and new beginnings. Goddess Durga is discussed further in Chapter 5, 'Chiron's in the House'.

As I moved through my initiation, I found the formidable force of these two Goddesses too strong at times and turned to the more soothing qualities of Goddess Lakshmi and Saraswati. Lakshmi stands in an ocean of milk, abundant, shimmering gold and rose, heralding a new dawn, peace, and joy. She's come through the battle and can rest in her bliss, soothing balm, faith, and satisfaction. Goddess Saraswati reigns over wisdom and creativity. She supports us in communication and eloquence, speaking our truth, with clarity, in a way that can be heard so it may be useful to invoke her during your menopause passage. You may also find other Goddesses that you resonate with that you wish to explore. Know that you can ask for help from these magnificent beings, invite them to support you on your initiation. This is explored further in Chapter 4, 'Who's in your Circle?'.

I have also suggested the use of mantra in some practices. Mantra is the repetition of sound vibration. The mantras are in Sanskrit, the ancient language of tantra and yoga and brings support, aligning us with the divine vibration in the manifest. When we chant mantra, our mind quietens, and we align with our inner being and the Divine. Sound is powerful and when used wisely, it uplifts us and changes the way we feel. It's like returning to our inner sound and fine-tuning our instrument. Mantra has been shared between one generation of seekers to another for hundreds of years. I have included the mantras of Goddess Kali, Durga, Saraswati, and Lakshmi as they hold the energy that I have most related to during my menopause. One of the lovely things about mantra is that no one need know you are practising. With silent repetition you can give the mind something to focus on wherever you are.

At times during this guide, I refer to the *chakras*. These are energy wheels or centres that are useful for our healing and bringing balance to our physical and energetic being. When we work with the chakras we can let go of old wounds and become more aligned with source or our higher selves. The chakras are related to the endocrine system, nerves, and organs. Our endocrine system secretes hormones that actively change the chemistry and physiological processes in our body. When we work with the chakras, we have a map of consciousness that communicates to us where we are out of balance or have blocked energy. The chakras have been used in yoga and tantra for thousands of years and other spiritual and esoteric systems also use these energy centres. They are also known as *interior stars*, which refer beautifully to our bodies being a microcosm of the whole cosmos, containing and expressing the planets and galaxies or *dragon jewels*. When we focus on balancing our chakras we can change our hormone functioning and over all well-being. This is particularly relevant to the menopause as the changes that occur are primarily hormone-based.

There are many chakras or energy centres in the body but there are six primary ones based within the spinal column. Each chakra embodies particular qualities or attributes, and we all have different *samskaras* or imprints that we hold in each. Part of our spiritual journey is to awaken and rebalance these energy centres. They are not as dense as flesh and bone so cannot be seen but as you become more sensitive and attuned you can feel them as energy. Each has associated, colour, vibrational sound and *bija* or seed mantra. Shakti energy, or *kundalini* lies coiled up at the base chakra often represented as a serpent. Through spiritual practice and awakening, this subtle energy rises through the chakras along the central column called *sushumna nadi*, piercing them to transcend these samskaras and allow the natural qualities of these abodes to flourish through us in our lives. Ultimately, this Shakti energy ascends to the crown of the head or *sahasrara*, uniting with unlimited consciousness beyond duality.

There are many excellent books explaining the chakras in detail, some of which are included in the bibliography. I will outline in brief in the Appendix 1 on page 159 as a preparation for some of the content within the following chapters, for those unfamiliar with the chakra system.

The rainbow is a powerful symbol and is a bridge from the cosmic energy to our manifest world. It holds the prism of light and vibration found in all things. It corresponds with the chakras system. It is no wonder that the sight of a rainbow brings such joy and spiritual nourishment. The practice of working with rainbow light can be useful, a rainbow meditation is included on page 108.

Menopause is a microcosm of the human condition. It is also a microcosm of this current time in our evolution and the evolution of planet earth. The earth is experiencing her menopause, as is humanity. We have enjoyed our 'summer', the sweet fertility, abundance of ideas, technological expansion, and skills. Now we feel and see the groans, pains of transformation and change. We don't need to look far to see this unfolding in our own lives and in the lives around us or on the news. In yoga this is referred to the age of *Kali Yuga* (Selbie & Steinmetz, 2011). The yugas are spans of time that transition in cycle. We have moved through the golden, silver, and bronze phases and are now in the iron span of time, which is considered a time of conflict and moral decline.

In traditional Indian life, there are four stages of life or *ashramas*. The first being that of learning, of living with a teacher. The second as householder, including job, marriage, and financial security. This is followed by retirement and a stepping back and letting go of responsibilities. The final stage is that of *sanyasa* where there is a renunciation of roles and identities. Worldly preoccupations are let go of and one's life takes on a spiritual focus. Although this is a traditional and non-Western cultural model, it resonates with the Western yogini or female spiritual seeker who is finding her way through her menopausal rite of passage. As we transition from our role as mothers, house keepers, carers, and continue careers into our crone years, we can choose to shift into a renewed focus, which can include spiritual focus, comprising a greater purpose than ourselves. Within Western culture such a spiritual dimension or phase of life is not acknowledged, encouraged, or supported. When we see our latter phase of life as time for personal integration and self-discovery we can perceive and engage with it from a place of curiosity, hope, and acceptance.

Ayurveda is the sister science to yoga and offers us much to support ourselves holistically. I have included some aspects of ayurveda in this guide, primarily with the focus on calming vata dosha. In Ayurveda, there are three doshas—vata, kapha, and pitta—and everyone has all three in varying degrees. They link to our constitution, including our personality and prevalent leanings. All the doshas have positive qualities but when they become out of balance, we can feel disharmony within ourselves. As we mature, we have a tendency to have increased vata. Vata is related to the element of air, it flows and moves and when out of balance can create anxiety, ungrounded feelings and erratic thoughts. Our society is predominantly vata at this time, with quick thought processes, a focus on electronics and moving quickly from one subject or object to another. So, vata can be even more heightened during our menopause. By incorporating some simple aspects of Ayurveda we can introduce more balance into our self-care.

Shamanism

Shamanism is an ancient tradition found cross-culturally which holds that Spirit or Source is in all things and all things are inter-connected. In shamanism, we work with benevolent spiritual guides or *tutelary spirits* to bring healing and guidance. This can often be in the form of animal guides who hold specific guidance and attributes for us to embrace. There are core shamanic healing techniques that help bring ourselves and our environment back into balance and harmony. In shamanism we shift our consciousness with intention from ordinary reality to non-ordinary reality where we can receive information and healing in connection with spirit guides. The shamanic state of consciousness offers a bridge between worlds or realities. This crossing through different states of consciousness is often referred to as moving through the *veil*. There are times where the veil is at its thinnest and we are more able to access and traverse these realities. One such time is the betwixt and between time of menopause.

When we consider the menopause as a profound spiritual shift, an initiation or rite of passage, we put it in a very different context to something that is a nuisance, best to be avoided, and to get through as quickly as possible. When we remember it is a sacred process, it can support us in surrendering a little more and having less resistance to whatever we are experiencing.

In shamanism, we can undergo a *dismemberment*, a healing journey that dismantles ourselves and then re-establishes us in a new way. This is akin to the menopause journey. There is a feeling that we are 'in pieces or bits' as we experience a fragmentation of our inner world or psyche. Visions and dreams are also an important part of the shamanic and wise woman path. I include several from my own experience to illustrate particular themes.

The use of ritual and ceremony are also important, and some chapters include suggestions for ritual and ceremony. Rituals are entered into with specific intention and take some form of structure. The contents of the ritual hold significance and symbolism, which can bring about transformation and healing for the individual or collective. Commonly, rituals include the four cardinal directions and acknowledgement of other beings that are called upon to support the ritual. Ceremonies mark a specific time or event, such as an opening or closing of a space or period of time or experience. The menopausal women can make good use of both of these to support her during her journey. In Chapter 8, I offer some ceremony suggestions that you can use or adapt to honour your menopause rite of passage.

Part of my shamanic journey has been with the Lyceum (Path of Pollen) a gynocentric shamanic tradition, which has its roots in Europe, including the Greek mystery schools. The Lyceum centres on the honeybee and the hive, a beautiful and potent matriarchal metaphor for our menopause. Within the hive the female workers work as a collective to bring harmony, health, and abundance to the colony. At the centre of the hive is the Queen, each Queen has her own essence, pheromones or flavour and the hive sings their song of contentment as they transform and transmute their foraging into an array of food, medicine, and protection for the whole hive.

Alchemy

The medieval alchemists and later, the psychoanalyst Jung, offered us a way to see psychological and physical processes as part of a transmutation. There are three main stages to the alchemical transformation, and each can be likened to the psychological and developmental stages of menopause. Alchemy observes and witnesses a change that occurs when two substances are brought together and a third or new stage is achieved. During our maturation process we integrate and assimilate different aspects of our personality and experience of the world. Our body is our alchemical vessel or *crucible* and holds this intense transformation process. When we hold this perspective, it shines a new light on symptoms and experiences. I integrate the sharings from a premise that our body is our vessel for alchemical change and transformation.

A woman's body is so awe-inspiring and yet, it is often taken for granted. Take a moment to marvel at how the womb is the vessel for new life, a container for forming and safekeeping of a new expression of source or Shakti. We have all had the delight of meeting a new baby and to be reminded of the pure bliss and radiance of being human and connected firmly to Source. It is part of the great mystery of life, we are the womb carriers, the creatrix, the Goddess incarnate. Notice how you respond when you read these words, perhaps you feel guarded, doubtful, or perhaps a remembering is ignited, a deep knowing and recognition.

The Change, as it is known, is moving towards more authenticity and of course this is not always wanted by those around us, so a circle of women who are experiencing similar experiences can be helpful or even a close friend. This can also be a time when investing time and money for yourself to have a neutral person to share with, such as a therapist or mentor who is aware of the menopause, can also be fruitful.

The initial alchemical stage is *nigredo* or black stage, we explore this further in the initial Chapters, 1, 2, and 3. This process is where the original substance is heated in fire and burnt to ashes. The second process *albedo*, the white stage, is explored in Chapter 5 and 6. This is where fluid is added to begin to bind what remains from the initial fire. The final stage is *rubedo* is the red gold stage. Here we see a new substance that was derived from the initial matter. We will explore this in Chapter 7 and 8.

Initiation

This book leans upon the framework of initiation as a reference point for our journey. All initiations have specific phases that are moved through, and the menopause journey takes us through those phases. These phases are cross-culturally recognised as initially separation, isolation, and severance, which is followed by transition, renunciation, and confrontation with death on some level. Finally, the initiate experiences rebirth, renewal, and return to the world. When we apply this process to our menopause passage it supports us in the process, it resonates so perfectly. I refer to these stages of spiritual initiation throughout the book as they relate to the stages that I and other women have experienced during menopause—*the big change, the transformer*.

The initiation phase of *separation* is marked in our perimenopause stage, where we begin to separate from what we have known and who we have been. We leave behind what is familiar in our lives and we are shaken up, things become different to how they were previously. This may be an internal shift or in external changes such as your relationship, job, or home. Usually, it will encompass several areas of your life. These themes are explored in Chapter 1 and 2.

Following this separation from what we knew, our identity begins to shift and an experience of unravelling occurs, we enter the *transition* stage. We experience being tested and challenged. This can feel brutal, lonely, and as if we are being pushed to our limits of endurance. This is particularly explored in Chapter 3, 'The Underworld' and Chapter 5, 'Chiron's in the House.' I have friends who are challenged by physical experiences and others who have huge financial, marital, and family challenges. Often this stage of initiation penetrates all aspects of our lives. It is a time of learning about ourselves, others, and our environment. It offers us a phase to re-access who we are and how our sense of self is expressed in the world. The inner and outer worlds may be at odds and in order for them to be redesigned and reassembled they first need to be dismantled.

This transition initiation stage is followed by the *return*. This is a time of integration and incorporating the newfound aspects of our experience. It is where we may make changes in our environment to align with the internal changes we have made. Prior to this, it can be hard to believe that there will be a return—we can experience fear that we will be left forever in a murky underworld. Yet, a second spring beckons, postmenopause. This is explored in Chapter 5, 'New threads Over Old' and following chapters.

Awareness of these different phases that you may experience can be helpful in navigating your way and can also support you getting a feel of when you need to express yourself, retreat, or mix with the world. The more you are able to listen to your intuition, inner guide, Source, the more clarity you will have about what you need at certain times. Throughout the book I will refer to Spirit in different ways, using these different terms. Essentially, I perceive it as all the same energy, and you can use the language that you prefer.

Although generally this book holds a positive perspective on this life phase, that is not to say that it is about denying, pretending, or putting a brave face on things. In contrast, it is about being authentic and becoming more aligned with our truth. For most women this is a testing and challenging time, most of us at some time or another will wish we could be drugged or even die, wanting to avoid the pain of initiation and transformation. I believe that most of us can hold both aspects, to hold a parallel experience, the ultimate multi-tasking, to hold both the pain and the hope.

Symptoms

When most of us think about the menopause we think of symptoms. This can have a negative connotation. The word 'symptom' is associated with Western medicine and the pharmaceuticals to manage them. Although I appreciate what Western medicine can offer and that it has supported many women, the term does not sit well for me in the context of conscious menopause. Throughout the book, I will mostly use the word 'experience' to encompass the emotional, mental, energetic, and physical 'symptoms' that can be experienced. Although this book will touch on some of the symptoms or experiences you may have during your menopause journey, this is not the book's focus.

There are many other excellent and widely available resources that you can access, some of which are included in the Further Resources section at the end of the book. In Chapter 8, 'Menopause Experiences and Welcome Relief', I have included some common experiences with suggested perspectives and practices that may support you. The list is far from complete, but I hope that it will be helpful. The suggestions made are helpful alongside consultation with your doctor and holistic practitioner. I have left a blank page for you to add any additional experiences, insights and ways you have found to bring relief that you can refer to in times of forgetting and to help guide other women.

There are several different types of hormone replacement therapy available and if this choice feels right for you, research which may be the best option for you. This book gives holistic alternatives to taking prescribed pharmaceutical medication. However, many women decide with full conscious awareness that this is the right path for them. We all have our own journey through this initiation and often the path of least resistance is the right option.

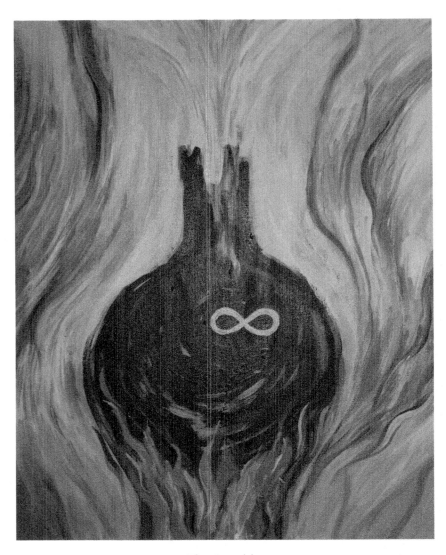

The Crucible

CHAPTER 1

Red River Runs Dry

As we move from our summer into our autumn phase of life, we experience perimenopause. This can start either naturally or be induced by having a hysterectomy or a sudden life change. I know of women who after the death of someone close to them began their menopause journey. This stage can be daunting, particularly as it is unclear when our final bleed will be.

Increasingly women are experiencing early menopause, this may be linked to several factors including stress, environmental pollutants and increased electronic usage. Alexandra Pope, founder of Red School and author of Wild Power (Pope, 2017), cautions that women in their 40s should not rush into the menopause but instead consider irregularities in their monthly cycle as a call for increased self-care. The forties can be a preparation for the menopause and if you have not previously attuned to the rhythm of your moon cycle this is a good time to start, even if your bleed is erratic.

I will give a brief overview here of the moon cycle map as I refer to this during the following chapters. Broadly speaking, the cycle can be likened to the seasons in nature. Each season corresponding to either the waxing or waning of the moon. During our inner spring, typically day five to eleven, we are like a new sapling, embodying the maiden energy.

Around day eleven we move into our inner summer and ovulation where we feel expansive and at ease. We then begin the decent into our inner autumn energies around day nineteen where we begin to turn inward. Following this, we transition into our inner winter and our bleed which is on day one of our cycle. Each woman is unique and what she experiences and when can vary. The menstrual cycle map offers a useful guide to support women during this phase of life. However, this changes as we enter perimenopause.

Perimenopause can be likened to the *separation* initiation phase. The feeling of things beginning to unravel begins and this can be frightening. We can try and hold on as best we can, keeping it all together, putting a smile on which becomes a grimace until finally we acknowledge that something has to change. It's a big shake up, things that used to help are no longer working—it starts to become clear that a new paradigm is needed. This emotional change and realisation can be a shock. It occurs as our monthly bleed also changes. This physical change can bring about huge feelings too. We are faced with reflecting upon our relationship with our monthly bleed.

I am a woman who began menstruating at age eleven and ended aged forty-nine. I had a gap of a few months for two pregnancies that were never carried to full term, but otherwise I had a regular cycle. That means I had about four hundred and fifty moon bleeds. That is a significant intimate relationship and therefore needs time and space to process and to reflect upon the change. Some of us liked our bleed and welcomed it, for others it felt like the 'curse' especially if symptoms were physically or emotionally debilitating. This relationship with your bleed will have a huge bearing on how you feel during perimenopause. There may be grief and there may be relief and all that sits in-between.

For some women the menstrual journey has been one of exploration and enquiry. Some of you will have consciously navigated your way through your cycle for some or part of your adult life. If you did so, there may be a feeling of a map having been taken away. If you enjoyed the surge of energy and creativity during the summer of your ovulation or relished the increased self-care, dream time, and rest prior to and during your bleed it can be experienced as a huge loss. One of the challenges is that we do not know when the last bleed will be. Perhaps you have been a woman that collects her blood and offered it to the garden, to the land or created with it as I did. This use of sacred fluid is now no longer available to you. It seems natural to have the final bleed so that it can be used in a rite of passage ceremony, but this may not be possible. This adds to a general feeling of uncertainty and feeling out of control.

For those of you who have followed your menstrual cycle, been conscious and aware of the rhythm and the seasons and moon in relation to your own unique rhythm, it can be quite a shock and destabilising when the bleed stops, an anchor point, an old friend departed. It is a salutary reminder of the depth of the menopause process when we realise that the menopause journey can be likened to being in your inner autumn and inner winter of your bleed for approximately ten years. It puts into perspective how it is so significant both to us and the people near us.

When you no longer have your personal menstrual map to guide you, either during erratic bleeding or once it has ceased, you can turn to the moon's own cycle as a guide. Awareness of the waxing and waning of her passage can offer a way to feel in-tune with nature's cycles and can offer some support. Again, every woman's process is unique and the change in bleed can be a gentle lessening, or it can involve flooding and pain that can be challenging in many ways. This is the time to use herbal supports alongside the perspectives and practices that I offer here. Susan Weed's book New Menopausal Years, Wise Woman Ways is an excellent resource.

Our bleed begins to change—the colour, texture, consistency, and regularity. It signals to us that things are moving towards an ending. For some women, this will be brought about abruptly, either through medical intervention, such as hysterectomy or trauma. Emotional change and external circumstances can affect our moon bleed. Sometimes we can think it is our last bleed only to have another bleed, sometimes for as long as a year afterwards. This can be disconcerting and confusing, another expression of how our world as we knew it is turned upside down.

If we are using contraception during this time, it may be more challenging to use, especially if working with natural methods. Like a fruit tree that has one last burst of abundance and creativity as it gifts huge amounts of fruit the season before it dies, the perimenopausal women can also have a last burst of fertility and attempt at conceiving. Many women are happy to become pregnant at this time but if that is not your desire then be mindful of the body's last surge to create life, adjust your precautions accordingly.

The cessation of our bleed means that we are no longer fertile in terms of giving birth to a baby. Our ovaries stop producing and releasing eggs which connect us to our animal self in a startling way. This marks finding ourselves at an axis in our lives that can feel shocking. Men can continue to be fertile into old age, yet women are faced with this junction. It is futile to deny, resist, or ignore. Here we begin to mourn not only the loss of our capacity to create human life but also to begin to face the reality that other things are also no longer possible. As we enter mid-life, we face in the direction of our mortality, our death, and the reality that there are some things we will never do in this life.

As women, we have been trained and conditioned by society to be accommodating to others' needs and orientate ourselves around others—parents, siblings, friends, partners, colleagues, children, and pets. I recall my good friend didn't have a weekend away for herself in fifteen years as she feared not being a good enough parent and partner and this is not uncommon. Men generally can make time for themselves and their own projects that nourish them and continue to maintain a sense of independence. Often, if women do, they hear the critical voice, whether spoken by another or internally from conditioning, of not being a good wife, mother etc. and this can lead to feelings of shame and fears of being judged as selfish. Women often carry the belief that to please others brings meaning to one's life.

The essence of the feminine is to be love and bring beauty to self, others, and environment (Odier, 1999). The feminine essence, or Shakti, is innately caring, generous, and harmonious but when this is not in balance with the masculine qualities of boundaries and stability we can become out of balance. If we have not already explored our need to have our own desires met and let go of the martyr archetype before the menopause, it can bring a startling realisation and shock that one has compassion fatigue and feels a bit pissed off that one's own needs have been disregarded for so long. Finding creative ways to explore and express these insights and feelings can be very helpful and help avoid long-term resentments and holding unexpressed emotions within the body. Arguably, it is these unexpressed and unmet needs and desires that can lead to imbalance and materialise as illness and disease. One can perceive breast cancer as being linked to the relentless care and giving to others that sucks a woman dry of her vital energy. This leads to the question; who am I without the roles that I've been playing?

If I was pushed, I would say that my perimenopause started around age forty-two. This is where the stirrings in my bones that something had to change couldn't be ignored. I had created a good life for myself; a stimulating and rewarding career as a psychotherapist. I could walk from my beautiful home along the river to get there, had lovely neighbours. I was on a good salary for doing what I had trained hard and long to qualify for, my work had meaning, and I supported others. I had good friends, worked part-time, and had a small private practice offering shamanic healing, a day in the pottery studio, kept bees and danced when I wanted. Despite all this, my whole being whispered and then screamed for change.

I had made a few adjustments: reducing hours, putting in more of what I love and that brings joy into my week and yet something still was a bit off. Perhaps some people in my position would have ridden it out, perhaps silencing or ignoring the unease, the growing dissatisfaction but I didn't have any dependents or anyone to answer to, so I left. I packed it all up. It was exciting and scary, but I felt a freedom in that leap and my friends supported me in doing so. It is interesting that when we take a leap of courage others are often happy to witness it. Perhaps they don't feel able to do it themselves, it's as if on some level you are doing it on behalf of others too.

In terms of the alchemical process, this is the black stage or *calcination*. The feelings of chaos, what had been previously hidden coming to light and our unconscious processes emerging, are all part of the perimenopause landscape. This shake-up phase and the underworld phase, explored in Chapter 4, mirror this alchemical process. Things that no longer serve us in our lives are thrown into the fire and burnt to ash.

The need to be alone can become huge, the whole system craving it and resenting any time when it is not possible. I recall experiencing any demands on me, even from people I liked and asking quite reasonable things such as listening to them, as feeling like an impingement. It was as if their need would stifle me and restrict me, I felt suffocated. The quest for self-orientation can become primary at this time. If this need for quiet retreat or depth of authentic communication is not met, one's fierceness and anger can escalate. It can be prudent, when the heat of this Kali or dark goddess energy is rising, for you to withdraw and find ways to harness or focus the energy. This can prevent expressing too much of the element of fire and its destructive qualities, to those around you or within your life.

Ideally, we have the resources to hold and care for ourselves, get the support we need and hold ourselves through this process. Or there may be someone that we can share this with, and they can hold us and support us through our journey. Shakti energy can take many forms. I like the phrase—*One Thousand Names of the Divine Mother*, as expressed in the chant the *Sri Lalita Sahasranama*. It acknowledges the many-faceted expressions of Shakti within embodied woman. We are at a time in our evolution that increasingly we can acknowledge all the faces or aspects of the Goddess—the fierce, loving, expansive, wise, compassionate, warrior, and so on. At this *calcination* stage she is in a wild state of raw energy, like the monsoon, earthquake, and forest fire. This powerful energy wants to be free, but it also can crave to be contained, to feel where the edges are. We will explore this further in Chapter 3, 'The Underworld'.

One of the ways that we can find an outlet for this energy is to have a fire. There can be a lot of fire, both heat in the body but also emotionally, during this time. This first alchemical process is known as the *Baptism of Fire* or *Nigredo* (Noack, 2017) and there is a lot of heat during this stage. One of the ways to give the element of fire an outlet is through deliberately having a fire. This could be a simple bonfire in the garden or a ritualised sacred fire. If you have a bonfire, you may also make it more ritualised by burning things from your past such as old letters or photos that you have held onto that you now feel ready to let go of.

The practice of vedic *agnihotra*, where a specific mantra is offered at the specific time of both sunrise and sunset, is a beautiful practice and has a purifying energy for ourselves and our environment. Another yogic fire is that of *havan*, which can be both powerful and supportive. A mantra is chosen and repeated a number of times (108 is traditional) and offerings are made to the fire or *agni*. For more information, please see Further Resources page 171. Using fire to transform energy with intention and mantra can be helpful at any time but particularly during menopause as it gives a sacred avenue and ritualises often intense and chaotic emotions, focusing them and transmuting them into an offering for a greater purpose. These sacred fires can be dedicated to the Goddess and intentions and resolutions can be made to support your process.

It is common during menopause to experience waves of intense anger and rage. Often this can be directed towards the masculine. We can uncover huge feelings of resentment towards the patriarchy, blaming them and ourselves for all the aspects of ourselves that have been oppressed and hidden. We can feel depleted from all the serving and caring if this has not been balanced with other aspects of ourselves such as self-nourishment and creativity. If we have had to comply and modify less acceptable faces of the Goddess within such as the wild, fierce aspects in order to receive conditional love, this can further stoke the fire.

In addition to the emotional and physical heat I also found my lack of enthusiasm quite disconcerting. The things that would normally spark my enthusiasm or interest me raised nothing—like a dead battery, no spark. Even friends or activities that I usually enjoyed slid by as I favoured a nice lie down in the dark. Once this had passed, it was easy to see it in the context of the journey, but at the time, like so many of the menopause experiences, it is shocking and concerning. Is this depression? Will I always feel like this now until I die? At times I would be bothered to try and focus my senses on something in nature, to look in wonder at an unfurling leaf, or the butterflies dancing together. Sometimes this helped and at other times it reinforced where I was. From here all we have is acceptance of what is and trust that a better feeling or thought will come again.

Anxieties about ageing and being less desirable can also begin to arise. We begin to feel different symptoms or experiences that are unknown to us. We can begin to fear becoming invisible, unnoticed, unseen. One woman shared her fear of becoming a 'nobody', a common fear.

In *Change of Life* (Mankowitz, 1984) Ann Mankowitz summarises the plight of the menopausal women within the context of societal perception …

> "… she is either insignificant, colourless, hovering on the periphery, hoping for a useful role, or she is flushed neurotic, moody as an adolescent but without the freshness or the promise."

Just as the menarche or the onset of menstruation marks the initiation stage from girl to womanhood, the last bleed marks our initiation towards our wise woman years. Often, we do not feel ready, there can be feelings of fear, regret, and sentimentality at what might have been. There can be a feeling, projected from social, religious, economic, and cultural conditioning, that as women we no longer have any standing in society once we are no longer of childbearing age. This coupled with the decline in our sexual power, can lead to feeling no longer valued, fearful and confused about our role in the world.

> "… our heroine is in a sad plight, faced with triple renunciation of youth, fertility and sexual power, and apparently, without any hope of rescue …" (Mankowitz, 1984)

At this time, we can identify with our physical womb, being no longer of use, dry and empty. This can connect with deep anxiety about living life never feeling fulfilled, that we will never experience the juice of life again.

It can be painful to acknowledge that we feel envy and jealousy towards our daughters and sisters for their youth and sexual power. The themes and emotions of envy and jealousy are still rarely spoken aloud, even in women's circles. Yet, acknowledge we must if we wish to look at ourselves clearly without distortion or gazing through the smeared glass of our mirror.

Contemplation questions

🪶 What do you need right now?

🪶 What has been your relationship with your menstrual cycle? Reflect upon how this may have changed throughout your life.

🪶 How do you feel about your bleed becoming irregular and then stopping? Perhaps this has already happened for you, if so, what are you still processing from this?

🪶 How can you express intense emotions in a way that is authentic but does not harm yourself or those around you?

🪶 What are the triggers to your intense feelings? Are there patterns that are familiar?

🪶 What hidden aspects of your personality in your unconscious are arising? How do you feel about meeting them?

Practices to support red river changes

Yoga nidra—crystal healing cave

Yoga nidra is a deep relaxation that is translated as *yogic sleep*. It is an excellent practice to assimilate changes, to balance and calm the nervous system and restore the mind and body, especially if you are having disrupted sleep.

For this practice, I suggest you read aloud the script and record it so you can use it when you wish. Read it in a clear voice at a steady pace.

Ensure that you won't be interrupted.

During the practice, I will refer to your *sankalpa*. A sankalpa is your resolve or intention, a short positive statement about your life that you will repeat several times during the practice. The seed of the sankalpa is planted in your unconscious, allowing it to flourish without resistance. Choose something that has real value and meaning to you before you begin the practice. A sankalpa is an affirming statement spoken in the present tense, for example: 'I am moving towards fulfilling my soul's purpose.'

To begin, lie in *shavasana* or semi-supine position. Allow a little space between your arms and the side of body and a space between the ankles. You may like to place a bolster or folded blanket beneath your knees or lower thighs.

Remove any bulky jewellery or glasses.

Set your intention to remain awake and aware during the practice.

Make any final adjustments to body or clothing. Allow the body to become still, only move if there is pain or significant discomfort.

Become aware of the connection between body and ground. All the parts of the body in connection with the body and ground. The feet, legs, buttocks, back, all the parts of the back, hands and arms, and the back of the head.

With every breath allow the body to become more relaxed and have a sense of letting go into the earth, knowing that she is supporting you and there is nothing for you to do but listen to the instructions.

Silently repeat your sankalpa, the positive affirming statement about your life. Repeat it several times with deep faith and conviction.

The next part of the practice is the rotation of awareness around the body. Follow my voice and as each part of the body is named, bring your awareness to that body part and mentally repeat the name of that part of the body.

Awareness to right hand ... right hand thumb ... second finger ... third finger ... fourth finger ... fifth finger ... palm of hand ... back of hand ... wrist ... forearm ... elbow ... upper arm ... right shoulder ... armpit ... side of body ... waist ... hip ... thigh ... knee ... back of knee ... shin ... calf ... heel ... top of right foot ... sole of foot ... big toe ... second toe ... third toe ... fourth toe ... fifth toe ...

Awareness now to left hand ... left hand thumb ... second finger ... third finger ... fourth finger ... fifth finger ... palm of hand ... back of hand ... wrist ... forearm ... elbow ... upper arm ... left shoulder ... armpit ... side of body ... waist ... hip ... thigh ... knee ... back of knee ... shin ... calf ... heel ... top of left foot ... sole of foot ... big toe ... second toe ... third toe ... fourth toe ... fifth toe ...

Awareness to right buttock … left buttock … lower back … middle back … upper back … the whole of the back … the spinal column … the whole of the back … back of neck … back of head … top of head … forehead … right temple … left temple … right ear … left ear … right eyebrow … left eyebrow … the space between the eyebrows … right eye … left eye … right cheek … left cheek … right nostril … left nostril … tip of nose … upper lip … lower lip … space where lips meet … tongue … teeth … chin … jaw … throat … right collar bone … left collar bone … right breast … left breast … centre of the chest … upper abdomen … lower abdomen … navel … the womb space … the elimination organs …

The whole of the right side of body … whole of left side of body … right and left side of body together … the front of body … back of body … front and back of the body together …the whole of the body … awareness of the whole of the body, whole body awareness …

Become aware now of your breath … the body breathing in and the body breathing out … begin to count the breath … count from the number twenty-seven downwards towards the number zero … inhale twenty-seven … exhale twenty-seven … inhale twenty-six … exhale twenty-six … continue in this way. If the mind wanders or you lose count of the breathe, just begin again from the number twenty-seven. Let go of awareness of the breathe and counting now, release counting the breath …

Become aware of the sensation of heaviness … allow the body to feel heavy. Surrender the whole body to the sensation of heaviness … heaviness in the feet … legs … hips … back … arms … and hands … the whole torso feeling so, so heavy … the head, and skull so heavy you can barely lift it … the whole body feeling heavier and heavier, as if made of stone … a dead weight … a heavy, heavy body … release the sensation of heaviness in the body now … fully let go of the sensation of a heavy body.

Allow yourself to experience the sensation now of a light body … the whole body feeling weightless and light … lightness in the fingers and toes, feet and hands … the arms and legs, so light they could lift off the ground … weightless body … torso feeling so, so light and the head and skull as light as a feather. Allow yourself to fully experience the sensation of a light body. Release the sensation of lightness in the body now … fully let go of the sensation of a weightless body.

Bring your awareness to the centre of the chest, the heart space, the activation point for anahat chakra. Allow yourself to breath here …

inhale into heart space ... exhale from anahat chakra ... continue this for several breaths. As you continue to breath, imagine or sense a flower at the heart space—as you inhale the flower expands, the petals unfolding ... as you exhale, allow the scent of this flower to fill your body. Continue in this way, breath after breath ... allow the scent and essence of this flower to fill your heart and whole being. After three minutes, release breath in the heart space. Now, let go of the flower.

Now bring the awareness to the dark space behind the eyes, the place of visions and dreams. I will say some images, use your imagination, visualisation, or sense them. Imagine you are walking along a coastal path ... you are aware of the vast blue sky above and the birds soaring above ... you notice the warm breeze against your skin ... as you continue to walk along the path you notice small flowers in the hedgerows, pink, purple, and white ... the path curves inland towards a rocky outcrop ... you begin to scramble over the rocks ... the rocks have absorbed the heat from the sun ... as you explore you notice an opening ... you decide to go inside ... it takes a moment for your eyes to adjust. As they do you see that you are standing inside a cave ... sunlight streams through a crack above and you see that the walls of the cave are covered in sparkling jewel-like crystals ... you look at the colours, shapes, and glimmering, shimmering stones, ingesting the beauty within ... you notice a small pool, the water is a milky turquoise ... you decide to explore the pool, undressing and allowing your body to sink into the warm water ... the pool seems to expand as you get in and you dive down to the bottom of the pool ... lying on the sandy bottom you are shown a symbol or object ... you know that this is offering you the guidance that you need at this time ... you bring the symbol or object towards your eyebrow centre ... then heart ... then ... womb ... ingesting the essence of this healing gift ... you give thanks to the pool, knowing it is time for you to return ... you swim upwards towards the light ... as you get ready to leave, you gaze once more at the shimmering healing crystals ... you express your gratitude towards the cave and leave ... you scramble back down onto the path and make your way back to where you began ...

Let go of this visualisation now ... bring the awareness to the heart space ... It is time for you to repeat your sankalpa once again, repeating it several times to yourself with faith and sincerity that it is manifesting in your life ... release your sankalpa now ... become aware of your whole body, the outline and physicality of your body ... know that the yoga nidra will soon be coming to an end ... become aware of the contact between floor and feet ... legs ... contact between the back and the ground ... the ground making contact with the arms and hands ... and the back of the head ... all the points of contact between body and ground ... become aware of the room that you are in ... noticing the body breathing and allow a couple of deeper breaths ... now that the yoga nidra is concluding ... continue to externalise your awareness ... gently allow the head to roll to one side then the other ... bring gentle movement to fingers and toes ... bring the knees up to the chest and give yourself a hug ... stretch and yawn ... when you are ready you can sit up ... take your time.

Spontaneous writing

Journal without censorship your thoughts and feelings about your relationship with your moon blood and feelings about it stopping.

Write a letter to your womb and ovaries, you might want to include how the relationship has felt, for example: distant, painful, intimate, appreciative. In your writing find some way to acknowledge that this is changing and express how you feel about that. You may wish to include acknowledgement of key events—for example, childbirth, start of menses, terminations, miscarriage, or not having conceived. If it feels right for you, express appreciation and gratitude.

Retreat

Prioritise retreat time. Depending on your life situation this may be a micro-retreat for fifteen minutes with an eye mask, lying on the couch, or twelve months on an island or in a woodland cave. However your life is at this time, be creative and find spaces for you to be alone and quiet.

Shaking

Shaking has been used cross-culturally in all spiritual traditions, including shamanic traditions and the Quaker, who literally quaked or shook as the Divine entered them. Shaking connects us with Source, brings healing, and shifts energy.

Stand upright with your feet slightly wider than hip width apart. Bring your awareness down to your feet, feel the connection with the earth beneath you. Feel gravity moving downwards through your body. Relax the face, soften the jaw and lips. Allow soft knees.

Begin to feel, imagine, or sense tremors in the feet, the movement rising up from the ground. Imagine that the energy is arising from the earth. Imagine an earthquake, if this helps; the earth naturally shaking, tremoring, and shuddering. Allow more breath as the shaking begins to increase in intensity, allow chaos to be expressed. Remember to look after your body, keeping the knees relaxed and soft. If the body does not wish to shake vigorously, focus on the shake being on the inside. Allow plenty of breath. Continue shaking for as long as feels right for you.

As you do so, trust the body to relax and shake in the way it needs to. Hold the intention to let go of any patterns of energy that are not useful to you and offer it to the earth. When you feel the shaking concluding, begin to slow down to stillness. Stand motionless and feel the life force energy, the Shakti or prana, circulating through the body.

If the body is hot and sweating, feel the sweat as healing nectar. You may like to rub it into your skin as nourishing healing balm. Breath in through the pores of the skin, imbibing the energy of your shaking practice.

Fire ritual to release the past

Collect the wood and light the fire. As it gets going, honour the fire by repeating out loud words that acknowledge the element of fire as a transformative element. For example,

I give thanks to the element of fire, I honour you in all your expressions, I ask that you transmute and transform my old habitual patterns of thinking/ behaviour/storyline.

Call in your guides and beings to support you (see Chapter 3, 'Who's in Your Circle?')

I give thanks to all Beings and ask that they step forward to support me in this ritual.

Speak aloud what you wish to release;

I ... (name) ... let go and release .... at this time. I give thanks for the role and place it has had in my life but now let go of it for the highest good so that I may step more fully into my authentic wise woman years.

You may also like to feed the fire with letters, poems, words, pictures that you have kept from the past, that express, symbolise, and represent things for you.

Allow the fire to consume what you have given.

Give your thanks.

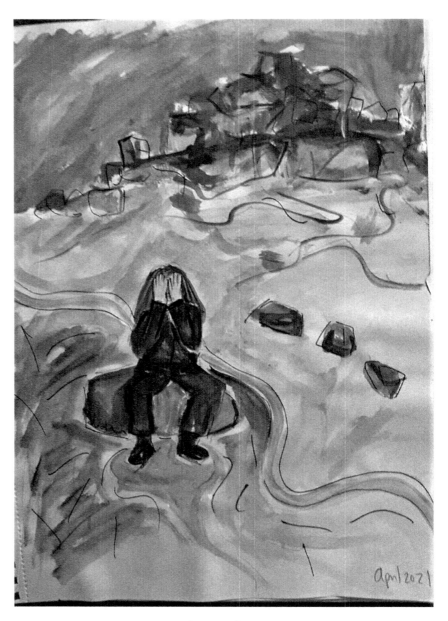

Red River Changes

CHAPTER 2

My Wild, Indigenous Body

Part of being conscious is to recognise that not only are we spiritual vibrational beings but that we also inhabit a sensory physical body. As we grow into maturation, part of the process is to integrate and balance these aspects. This is likened to the alchemists bringing together different substances to integrate through *coniunctio* or the conjunction of opposites.

In our experience as a civilised human being, we can forget and grow apart from the fact that we are embodied natural beings. Dogmatic religion and some spiritual traditions may steer us away from honouring our bodies as expression of the Divine. We are part of nature, not separate from it, our animal selves need to be honoured and recognised. As society attempts to tame and restrict the expression of our free animal selves, these aspects can become distorted and denied. This often leads to perverse expressions of our untamed, unaccepted, and unacknowledged parts. This can then find expression in behaviours, such as sexual abuse and violence. As we grow up from baby to toddler, child, teenager, and young adult, we learn the attitudes and behaviours that are expected from us. We conform because we want to be loved and accepted. There are conditions around receiving this love and acceptance, and most of us weigh up whether it is worth the cost of squishing, adapting, and making aspects of ourselves smaller or bigger to receive this conditioned love and acceptance.

The desire to touch and be touched whether by another human, by nature or by ourselves is natural and healthy. Many spiritual paths including tantra, recognise this and advocate and encourage us to embrace all aspects of ourselves, including our physicality. This also includes our emotional aspects; the passionate, angry, jealous, trivial, judgemental, longing for recognition, and shameful aspects. It can be an important part of our conscious menopause to make a practice of not denying our worldly sensory desires, our bodies and our unwanted shadow aspects. As we shine the light of awareness on how we really are in any moment we begin to accept ourselves and others more fully. The sensual body and senses are not an inconvenience to our path but a gateway to deeper connection with source. Odier explains that our body has deep knowing and that as we become truly present to reality via our interaction with the world, we experience the tremor of consciousness and no longer feel that something is missing. (Odier, 1999)

When we take time to bring our awareness to present moment reality, we can shift our consciousness and experience ease and spaciousness. Often, we have split energy and awareness. Notice what you are doing when you are doing it, how your body moves, what you can hear, when you eat, the sensations on your skin from touch, how your eyes absorb the world around you. It is usual for the mind to interpret or fictitiously create a narrative of your experience, but if we can just be and relax, we can find an oasis of stillness and ease.

For many of us, the reality is that to fully embrace ourselves there first needs to be an unpicking and an unravelling of what we have been taught. Some of us were taught not to enjoy our bodies, not to touch ourselves for pleasure or revel in the delight of touch. When I say self-pleasure and touch, the mind tends to leap to masturbation. In our society, touch is equated to sexual pleasure and the pornography industry and media have both encouraged and profited from this. Sensory pleasure is rarely acknowledged and yet it is this sensory pleasure (whether sexual or not) that can lead to an experience of connection and contentment.

Some of us have journeyed to adulthood with many perceptions of how we need to behave, many of the conditions that we inherit are related to our relationship with our bodies. There can be tremendous freedom when we can release the grasp that some of these rules and conditions have had on us. We can reach menopause and find ourselves saying 'hang on a minute, it makes no difference to how I experience the world whether I do what I like, or I try and second guess what others want of me'.

One of the experiences I have had at significant turning points in my life, including menopause, was of feeling confined, as if my skin was too tight. The analogy of the caterpillar in a cocoon comes to mind. It's as if one has grown and expanded and is now too tight in what was previously a protective environment. What was once protective now feels restrictive, perhaps even suffocating. What was once comfortable has been outgrown. Yet it is not possible to move out of this cocoon if it is not ready. There is a limbo phase, a time when you are neither caterpillar nor butterfly. This is particularly the case during pre- or perimenopause.

These in-between phases can be extremely challenging. They are the between and betwixt places of dusk, twilight, dawn and midnight, the places where the Dark Goddess likes to hang out and where the alchemist knows anything is possible. This is the place of the menopausal woman. It may not feel like it at the time, but these crossroads and junctions are potent transition spaces where day turns to night and night to day. These in-between places are recognised in many spiritual traditions as significant, the liminal non-linear spaces that are neither one nor the other.

When I was feeling like this, I would sometimes feel impatient, knowing that I needed to expand but not being able to. I would walk beside the lake where I lived and sit on the grass, watching the horses and goats moving about their day unfazed. During a particular phase, a heron would often be there, sitting very still. Sometimes I would disturb it and it would take off, its amazing wingspan spreading into the sky only to settle again a little further away in complete stillness. She was waiting, waiting and then waiting some more. I realised that this was the teaching, or gift, from the heron to me, to be patient and wait. The heron does not push or grasp but waits for the fish to come to her. The heron clearly demonstrated that patience is rewarded with abundance and golden fish.

Several months after my encounter with the heron I read Sharon Blackie's *Chronicles of Old Crane Woman* (Blackie, 2022). She writes that in Irish mythology the heron and crane are interchangeable. She says that they are associated with longevity and in some of the old stories they are connected to hags and old women.

"In those old stories, crane is a powerful and a liminal bird. She haunts the thresholds where water, land and air intermingle; she guards the treasures of the Otherworld and is a guide to those who wish to travel there ... she is associated with shapeshifting in the feminine form ..."

This feeling of waiting became more palatable as I explored ways to feel freedom from within, to be open to spaciousness through meditation, intuitive dance and movement. I would wriggle, sway, and move as if beginning to ready myself to wriggle out of my cocoon. Does the caterpillar know it is waiting to become a butterfly? Perhaps not. In the same way we do not know what is on the other side of the menopausal rite of passage. In the waiting period, we are blind, we rely on a natural organic process, we trust and hold onto the knowing, however tentative, that we are in a process of transformation. We have stepped into the initiation phase of *transition* and something is happening that will mean we will be different afterwards.

Down in the woods I would enjoy exploring the wildness, the untouched areas. Moving with awareness through the brambles, ferns, and trees. I would pause, listen, wait, and absorb. Ingesting the wildness of nature, not the tamed, manicured, and restricted parts of nature, the gravel paths and pruning, but feeling and connecting into the wildness and seeming chaos. Absorbing the energies from the plants and earth through skin and breath.

One way to connect quickly with the earth energies, to ground ourselves and reconnect with our indigenous selves is by walking barefoot. This practice is so available, easy, and accessible and yet uncommon. Many of us have forgotten how important it is to connect with the vibrations of the earth and that wearing rubber soles cuts us off from and distorts the energies, keeping us removed and ungrounded. Women, and men, who experience symptoms that signal a need for re-balance, whether emotional, mental, or physical ill health, can find significant relief from this simple practice.

In Ayurveda, the menopausal time of life is associated with the *vata dosha*[2], as we get older the vata dosha increases (Lewin, 2017). Qualities

---

[2] In ayurveda there are three doshas or constitutional types—vata, pitta, and kapha. Vata dosha is prominent in our society and in menopause. By soothing and calming vata dosha we can bring ourselves into balance.

of this air element include quick thought processes, lack of concentration and a susceptibility to feeling ungrounded or uprooted. The more we can keep our vata in balance the easier and better we will feel. Walking barefoot can be a simple yet effective way to balance ourselves and vata dosha.

Being bare foot is just one part of this reconnection with one's wild and indigenous self. Many of us are only naked when we shower or make love. Often, we have a lot of conditioning around nakedness. Our society has distorted nakedness to being about sex; many women and men feel unsafe being naked with others in a non-sexual context. How far are we removed from our wild, natural selves? When you go to the beach, you may see a toddler with no self-consciousness of their nakedness, exploring the sea for the first time with support from a parent. We are reminded of the ease we felt as a child in our bodies and the acceptance of the world around us. This freedom in our bodies is quickly lost as we grow up, along with freedom of movement and expression. Adults can predominantly sit still talking or chatting, even if physically and/or emotionally uncomfortable, for several hours, yet a child will intuitively move around their space, following their inner energy and natural desire. It can take time to let go of our old, conditioned responses around our bodies and in particular nakedness. We often need to reconsider our boundaries and our sense of choice, and this can help us develop increased feelings of safety and trust.

For most women, the experience of being bare-breasted is for brief moments every day; in the shower, changing clothes, making love, breast feeding. This is very different for men. Men almost have permission from general society to be bare-chested whenever they wish, when feeling hot or working outdoors. Perhaps, simply because they wish to feel the element of air on the skin, the warmth of the sun on their nipples, or lie on the ground and feel the soil and tickle of the grass beneath them. This is not the case for women. This is likely to relate to the sexual objectifying of women's breasts, that they are consciously or unconsciously perceived as objects for male pleasure. Despite increased equality between the sexes, this has increased over the last few decades even to the extent that breastfeeding in public is prohibited or scorned upon. Such contracted and distorted perceptions about this part of the body have led to a perception of our breasts as being separate from our whole being and subtly communicates that they do not belong to the women themselves. When the natural expression and freedom of anything is not permitted and, in this case, our breasts, the natural flow of energy is blocked, leading to stagnation, illness, and disease.

There can be shame attached to being bare-breasted, a huge distortion from our natural, indigenous, and authentic self. During menopause we are invited to deepen our relationship with our whole body which includes our breasts. Through touch, massage, and self-awareness of associated feelings and sensations we can begin to experience the breast as an instrument that can tune into non-cognitive and rational thinking beyond the veil and seek out the liminal spaces. We can be open to the possibility of deeper sensory communion with the elements around us.

In menopause, we can become aware of our breasts changing shape and function and this can be emotive and challenging. We may feel self-conscious, less desirable, and fearful of judgement. When we have courage to explore being bare-breasted outside the usual permitted confines it can be a significant experience and depends on our family and cultural conditioning. There can be a huge feeling of vulnerability. The breasts are such a sensitive part of our body, one step is to be bare-breasted with ourselves, another, with other women and then another step to be bare-breasted with both men and women. If we observe thoughts and feelings that arise, it may be surprising to witness the insecurities that underlie this. Ranging from fear to comparisons and insecurities about breast size or shape. There may also be fear of unwanted sexual attention and even sexual violence. For some women, it can also trigger memories and flash backs related to previous sexual trauma.

It is fascinating and refreshing when we consider breasts as being sensitive, receptive, and potentially powerful organs or receptive instruments. Just as the fine hairs on our skin and hair on our head act as antennae, picking up vibrations from the world around us, our breasts can also tune into natural vibrations and bring us information. In some priestess or Shakti traditions the breast and nipples were, and are, regarded as a divination tool. Through certain esoteric practices the breasts are used to drink deep, drawing up information from Source to feed and nourish oneself and the community. The old phrase 'as pointed as a witch's tit' is potent as this is likely to refer to a time when a wise woman would use their breast to point and divine wisdom, tapping into the knowledge in the earth's veins. Our breasts therefore do not need only to provide mothers' milk to baby but this gift can extend to feed and nourish a whole community with guidance and prophecy.

On the land where I lived, we would have regular oak wood-fired saunas and monthly sweat lodges on the night of the dark moon, where women and men would be naked together. Other times, we would work naked, on the land together. Sometimes I felt acutely self-conscious and vulnerable and at other times it felt liberating, natural, and beautiful. It was so enjoyable collecting twigs for kindling by myself, in the wild wood, wearing nothing but wellies and a hessian sack slung over my shoulder.

I remember when I first arrived on the land, I was asked to cut some reeds to put on the floor of the sweat lodge. A special type of reed that is found in marshy areas, it is a plant usually regarded as useless and unwanted. Yet, they have incredible natural insulation and padding and have been used for centuries for carpeting our dwellings and for sleeping on. Another member of the community was helping me, he is a man of presence and had been living on the land for a while and was incredibly muscular and naked. Apart from the occasional sauna or ceremony, I had never been naked with a man unless during sexual intimacy, so it was newish territory. So off we went with our bread knives and nakedness bending over cutting reeds together sharing our life stories. It was a sweet introduction, and I was faced with my own preconceptions, judgements, and sexual boundaries.

Sadly, not everyone can explore this in their immediate environment, but we can all explore our own perceptions and explore nudity for the sheer pleasure of it and have increased awareness in our own homes. Allowing the skin to feel the different sensations and temperatures of air is a wonderful way to bring us into the here and now.

This is also true with our connection to water. Many women find that wild swimming feels good during menopause. I have had beautiful moments where I have been birthed out of the sweat lodge and made my way down to the natural pool and river, like a baby turtle searching for the sea, and submerged myself in the cold water under the stars. Being immersed in water can feel very supportive and spacious. The exhilaration of the coldness hitting the system can help the nervous system and some women swear by it for assisting inflammation and brain fog. Pools, rivers, the sea, any reservoir body of water can allow us to connect with our own water bodies and depths of unconscious. It can also be part of purification and cleansing. Many women also find that wild swimming really helps with symptoms and experience coming back to themselves, the energy of the sea particularly allows us to replenish and renew our own energy field. There has been recent research showing the positive effects of wild swimming on the nervous system (Gifford, 2022). It allows us to connect with the vast ocean and her wildness and reminds us of the ebb and flow and continuous wave of our own lives. A river or sea does not remain static, she is constantly changing, an expression of Shakti just as we are. It is reassuring and validating, any body of water reflects to us our own true nature. When we swim wild or explore being unclothed, we allow ourselves to meet the unusual, an edge or discomfort, we play on the boundary of our comfort zone. This boundary is where transformation occurs.

As a woman, one of our most powerful ways to feel grounded and connected to Source is through our yoni. Our womb space is a source of great wisdom and power. The womb is the vessel of birth, new life and creativity. As we begin to place more awareness on this, we begin to receive feedback, we begin to experience the capacity of the womb space and yoni as a sacred vessel or cauldron. In the Lyceum, a European gynocentric shamanic path, the yoni is referred to as the *'first brain'* and in this path it is encouraged to allow your first brain to guide you in your thought, speech, and action. Daniel Odier describes the Shakti traditions and that in the scripture *Yoni Tantra* it says, 'The yoni is worshipped as the dwelling place of the goddess.' (Odier, 2016)

This source of power and information is actively closed off in our society. One of the ways that this is reinforced is by the wearing of underwear all or most of the time. This creates a block and a separation from our connection with the earth energies. It is liberating to go about your day without underwear. A long, thick full skirt is ideal for this, especially in colder climates. This is how many of our ancestors would have lived. Being knickerless allows a direct energy pathway between the earth's energy, our Mother, and your body, in particular your womb space. Through this connection between earth energy and womb space we can nourish our own energy and feed the creative vessel. Through doing so, we open ourselves up to receive inspiration and ideas that can then be birthed and manifested into reality. We can also ensure we are replenished and not 'sucked dry' by others needing our love and care.

I recall a woman who attended a sacred feminine workshop I facilitated. As part of this retreat we danced freely and ecstatically. I invited the women to take off their underwear and, if they wished, hang it on the surrounding trees. Afterwards one woman told me that it had felt enormously liberating as she always wore underwear, even when in bed. This is a poignant example of how habitual it has become to close ourselves off from our connection to our yoni and to the energy of the earth.

One of the best things about not wearing any underwear is that you can pee outside (wild wee) whilst standing up. This experience is very different from squatting. This is also easily done if naked outside. Peeing standing up can also be done in the bathroom with a standard loo too. It is empowering and liberating, perhaps because it creates a golden thread or stream between body and earth. It also encourages you to stand in the Goddess pose which is grounding, strong, and expansive.

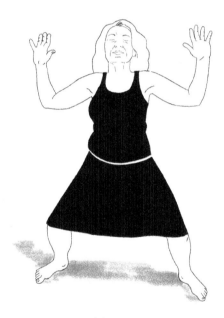

Goddess pose

In this phase during our menopause, we begin to let go of our inauthentic selves, our conditioned roles. This is likened to the alchemical phase of where the old structure is being dismantled and broken down by the fire, to leave ash and dust. In the purifying yogic practice of *agni-hotri*, the ash is considered sacred and rather than being discarded as a waste product it is respectfully saved and used as medicine for ourselves, animals, plants and soil. What makes it sacred and healing are several factors including the mantra that is recited, but perhaps more

importantly it is the focused intention during the practice and the transformative nature of the fire. This ash can be used in our water, food, and
gardens.

Whilst in the wood, I connected to huge amounts of grief, not only in
relation to environmental changes but also because of how rare it is for
a human to feel wild and indigenous. Although I lived in eighty acres
of untamed woodland, pasture, and meadowland, the land was surrounded by managed agricultural land. Strange, foreign noises could be
heard from nearby farms. During one dark moon retreat I connected to
my own indigenous wild self, and I began to have a sense of what other
indigenous people must experience. The sounds nearby; of logging,
trailers, machinery, unknown voices made me feel uncertain of what
was happening, how close they were or what they were doing. In this
mind state, it was easy to feel unsafe, unsettled, unsure, and defensive,
and wonder if my space and environment were in danger and potentially threatened. This experience led me to contemplate, 'what would I
do to protect my home and pristine, natural environment?' Walk away?
Fight? At these times we are faced with evaluating what really matters.
We are also faced with the reality that we too are the protagonists and
the perpetrators. Our menopause asks us to reflect on what is important
for us, when to walk away and when to fight for what we believe. This
process can help us to have more clarity about life, our impact on others
and our environment, and avoid wasting energy.

Like many of us I was brought up by parents who were post-war
babies, their parents had been managing the aftermath of war and a
sense of scarcity was prevalent. People were cautious. My parents
worked hard and were very aware of the perceptions of others, it was
important not to make a scene or attract unwanted attention to yourself. Generally, women did not talk about their menstrual cycle or the
menopause. Creative expression such as dancing, singing, or any other
spontaneous action was usually regarded as showing off and discouraged, unless done so within an acceptable framework. Strong emotions and displays of those emotions were also discouraged and met
with concern and confusion. Such reflections are not about blame but
rather an enquiry and an acceptance of our influences. This acceptance
and understanding of our parents, guardians and culture can grow
into gratitude and appreciation, an important phase in our maturation
whether in menopause or before.

My wild, indigenous self was tamed, clipped, and shaped as most of us have been. Gradually during my late teens and young adulthood, I began to explore, primarily through expressive art making and free ecstatic dance, I began to make a mess. Through art making, I had the permission to feel into my silenced chaos and express unconscious and hidden aspects of myself. Gabrielle Roth's 5 Rhythms ecstatic dance and other expressive intuitive dance, movement, and voice work were also major vehicles for this. Allowing ourselves to express and create beyond given guidance, predetermined steps, rules, or boundaries can open up a rich landscape. After many years, I finally reconnected to my body and had permission to move with abandon, from the inside out. Similarly, shamanic work gave permission for the expression of sound, imagination, and hidden intuitive aspects to have a space to shine and develop. We all have our own stories and pathways, the crafted routes, streams, and threads that we have traversed to come more and more into balance. The menopause gives us another opportunity to tend to these hidden aspects and fine-tune what has already been re-found and integrated.

Whether barefoot, knickerless, or bare-breasted, we open our intuitive faculties, waiting and being open to being led by our body rather than from a head place. Such things in our culture can attract a lot of judgement. Our minds can quickly access labels such as being 'loose, easy, and asking for it'. If we choose to explore these avenues towards wholeness of expression, it is important that we are gentle with ourselves, softening to our own pace and having time and space to process what may arise in our exploration. These labels prevent women from connecting to their innate power, wisdom, and sensitivity. When we honour and experiment with these, even if in your own home, we can expand our awareness, perception, and connection to source. These practices can bring a sense of freedom, autonomy and spaciousness, which can be a welcome balm during our menopausal passage.

Our bodies are our alchemical vessel, and the honeybees and bee mystery schools know this. The bee is a sacred ally in many spiritual traditions, including the Lyceum. The honey bee teaches us the miraculous capacity of the body to transmute substances and create healing *nektars* (Buxton, 2004). Through the foraging of natural matter, such as tree resin, pollen, water, bees create food for their young and the community, royal jelly for their Queen, medicine, and protection for the community. The bees transmute through an internal alchemy a particular base matter into another product that is needed by the colony. Similarly, substances created by our bodies, such as urine, sweat, and menstrual blood, can be transmuted through certain practices into medicine. Like humans the increase in use of pesticides, the reduction of wild nature and increase in technology has caused a huge threat to their communities. The beehive is a matriarchal based community, they work as one mind, flowing and adapting to what is needed by the community at any given time. Colony collapse disorder (CCD) has seen a huge number of colonies' demise in recent years. Like the humble honeybee we have the capacity to heal ourselves and others through our intention and harnessing the energies of the natural world around us.

The wild woman can be found in the spaces, edges, and the unknown territory of our lives. If you haven't met your wild woman much before, you can encourage yourself to go off the known path, move in unfamiliar ways, and do things at times which you might never have done before. Perhaps a walk naked under the light of the full moon, moving in uncensored ways, and uttering sounds without meaning. If we give ourselves permission, things can start to shift, creativity and spontaneity become more accessible. With this wild woman energy, we can loosen and wriggle free from outgrown, stuck places and maintain the capacity to change and flow with life, creating agility in body and mind that is less willing to calcify and become rigid.

Contemplation questions

How do you feel towards your wild, indigenous self?

What messages have you been given during your life about being wild?

In what ways does your body communicate to you about whether it is satisfied or not in its depth of expression?

In what ways do you feel contracted and how does this state express itself in the world?

What thoughts and feelings arise when you walk bare-footed?

What thoughts and feelings arise when you choose not to wear underwear outside the usual situations?

What thoughts and feelings arise when you are bare-breasted? (With yourself, other women, with men and women.) Does your relationship with your breasts have a different quality when outside the usual situations?

What thoughts, feelings, and associations arise when you are naked outside the usual situations?

How can you honour and give your wild woman more space to express herself?

Practices to awaken and support your wild woman

Circular yoni breath[3]

Lie comfortably on the floor. Have your knees bent and feet more than hip width apart, support yourself with your elbows. If this is not comfortable you can use stacked pillows or lean against a wall.

Become aware of your mouth and release any holding or tension in the lips and jaw. Open your upper mouth gently, softening lips, as you do this notice the correlation with your lower lips. Become aware of your lower yoni lips and release any holding or tension.

Using your intention and imagination, breathe in through your yoni and out through the mouth. If able to do this naked, bare-breasted or in nature, bring awareness to what these different experiences bring.

Continue with natural breath without straining or pushing, inhaling through yoni, exhaling through upper mouth, become aware of the circular motion of the breath. Complete awareness of the energy moving around in a circle through your body.

Once you have established this you can explore breathing in the other direction. Inhaling through the upper mouth and exhaling through the lower mouth.

---

[3] Circular Yoni Breath is a practice known as *Labiomancy* as taught in the Lyceum tradition.

The next stage of the practice is to explore using a quality or aspect from nature. Using your imagination, sensing or visualising you can practice the circular yoni breath whilst using the spring green colour of the hawthorn tree, the warmth of the sun rising, or the earthy smell of soil following the rain. There are countless qualities you can work with, choose the natural essence that you need at any particular time. For example, you may feel you wish to imbue the healing resin of propolis into your aching body, ask the bees for their support. Imagine the smell and quality of this resin as you breathe or you may wish to practice with the quality of a cooling stream if you are experiencing a lot of heat.

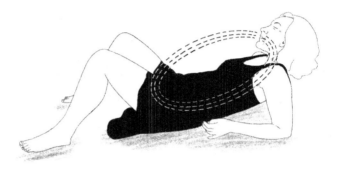

Circular yoni breath

Intuitive movement and sound

Either to music you may not usually listen to or to the sounds of nature or the environment around you, begin to give the body permission to move.

Allow the movement to come from the inside out, listen and feel from the inside, connecting to your breath and body.

Set your intention to follow how your body wishes to move, this may be slow and sensual or rhythmic and fast.

If sounds choose to arise, then allow them to come. Keep returning and connecting to your centre and allow the body to lead.

This practice can reveal beautiful surprises and can lead to expression and release of emotion that may be otherwise difficult to access. Spontaneous movement and sound can take you by surprise and allow different thoughts to flow through the unfolding of creative intuitive expression.

This practice may last ten minutes or an hour depending on the time you have available. At the end, be still and become aware of how you feel physically, emotionally, and mentally.

Walking barefoot

As you walk barefoot become aware of the sensations under foot such as heat, coolness, dry, soft, or damp.

Awareness of placing your heal down on the ground first, then the side, followed by the front part of the foot and toes.

You may like to slow your walking down, so that every step is pregnant with awareness.

Bring awareness to the soles of your feet and know that the soles are receptors. Allow them to inhale the earth energies into your whole being.

As you do so, know that you are taking in nourishment from the earth and as you exhale through the feet allow yourself to release what is no longer wanted or needed. This could be an emotion such as fear, anger, or jealousy or even a physical experience that you are struggling with, such as vertigo.

Earth scratching

Lie on your back, knees bent, arms at the sides of your body. Feel yourself supported by the earth.

Ensure the jaw and mouth are relaxed and become aware of your natural breath.

Begin to allow your hands and feet to move against the earth, allow the fingers and toes to begin to scratch and claw at the earth. Allow the rest of the body to follow as it wishes. As you move allow plenty of breath and allow any sounds to come that arise. Begin to exaggerate the movement, if it feels right, allow the body to writhe and growl, be aware of your sense of smell and touch.

When it feels time to finish, slow down the movement and then become still.

Become aware of the sensations you feel and the life force flowing through your body.

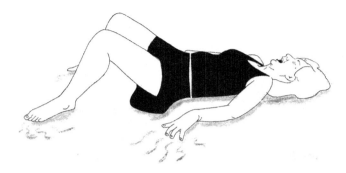

Earth scratching

Breast massage

Make sure you are warm and have some oil that pleases you, perhaps olive oil mixed with an essential oil such as lavender or frankincense. Begin by warming the oil. This can be done by standing a container of oil in a bowl of hot water for a few minutes.

Either sitting or lying down, inhale, breathing energy down through the crown of the head to the breasts and up from the earth. As you exhale allow these energies to meet and expand into the breasts. Feel the nourishing energy. Continue for several minutes.

Warm your hands and coat them in oil. Stroke the infinity symbol, figure of eight, around the breasts several times, then pause and move in the other direction.

Smooth the oil over the breasts in circular motions, towards the heart and then away from the heart. Feel the sensation, bring as much awareness as possible into the sensation you are feeling.

There are many nerve endings in the breasts, especially in the nipples. Gently pull the nipples, feel the aliveness, the response in the whole body.

Continue to explore different touch and sensations whilst holding an attitude of love and acceptance.

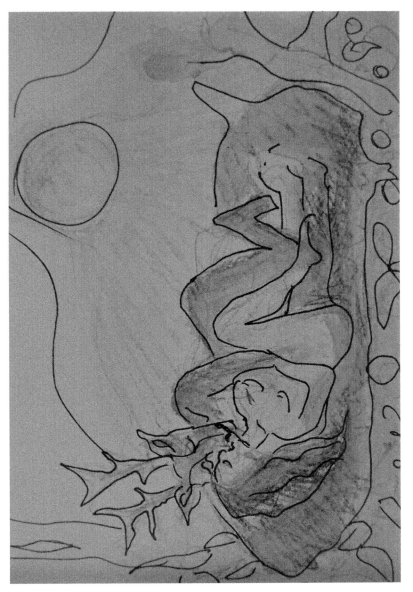

With Pan

CHAPTER 3

The Underworld

At the peak of the initiation process comes the death phase, the 'shake up' that we explored in Chapter 1, which shifts into a dismantling of the self. It allows the old way and old egoic identity to be loosened enough for there to be a giving up and a surrender. This can be met with great despair or feeling overwhelmed at the uncertainty of life. We might have had clarity about life and our purpose in it, perhaps as a mother, or in a profession and now we can feel very unstable, fragile, and precarious. Here we writhe in the black stage of our alchemical process.

In our society, this notion of letting go can be seen as a negative trait; we live in a culture whereby following one's inner energy is unacceptable. To sleep in the afternoon or to wail like a banshee is strongly discouraged and can illicit responses such as 'pull yourself together'. When we attend to our own soul needs, it is often perceived as selfish. And it is, we are responding to our soul's deep need and desire, and it is self-orientated because it needs to be. Yet, not letting go or honouring our inner journey can be deeply detrimental to ourselves and to those around us. The supressed and denied longings of expression in our lives can become stagnant energy that evolves into imbalance and eventual dis-ease, which can take the form of physical and mental illness, such as cancer and depression. It is a paradox that when we do attend to our own needs, we can live a more vibrant life and be more available to those we share life with. An example of this is the analogy of the pre-flight safety demonstration that instructs us to put on our own oxygen mask before helping a child, illustrating this beautifully.

During the menopause, all of our emotions that we have modified, denied, and ignored, can scream out for attention. They are not willing to be mollified, muffled, and diluted, and there is a new refusal to comply. It is as if an appropriate societal filter is removed and what previously we would have left unexpressed or perhaps conformed to, now, it is no longer satisfactory to do so. These emotions want to be heard. It can be an intense time and if we choose to resist, it may mean that these symptoms are more intense and continue for longer. Alternatively, we have the option to surrender and navigate the journey as best as we can.

This phase is often described as the *dark night of the soul* (Haas, 2018). It can be experienced as a spiritual crisis when the yearning of the soul wants to move to the front of the line. It is a sacred crossroads. Here, we can feel powerless, empty, fearful, and uncertain. When our usual coping strategies no longer serve us, and we are unable to find comfort from ourselves or others we may even contemplate suicide. Either symbolically or literally, time is spent in a tomb or grave and this stage is common to all initiation rites. As with other significant life passages, from a soul level we chose when we begin the journey, the timing and the how, including the menopause.

As we journey deeper into our menopausal journey, we descend deeper into the underworld. The underworld is included in many myths in all traditions. This world below the living world is often referred to as a place of quests and challenging journeys for the heroine or hero. It is the realm of death and souls. With the descent we are challenged, ourselves vulnerable and stripped bare, our soul's quest or inner self is our compass.

We have a choice in menopause whether to resist the invitation to face our shadow or to drop into the void of unknown territory and acknowledge that this is where we are, and we can ride the wave as best as we can. This wild ride can require a wild rider, and if we invoke our wild woman, it can be so positive. She knows how to lie in the tomb and grieve what has been lost. She knows how to dance barefoot on the earth under the dark moon, offering with every step her anger, tears, and bitterness to the earth. We are in a process of remembering.

During this time old random memories may pop up like a surreal theatre show with their associated pains. Cruelty, loss, and heartbreak, emotions you thought you had dealt with begin to rear their ugly heads again. Ugly they may be, but they come with an invitation. An invitation to face head on, delve even deeper, illuminate, be with, chew over or spit out.

One of the emotions that arises is grief. There are so many layers of grief within us; people that are no longer in our lives, either through change or death, grief for lost dreams and missed opportunities. We mourn the fruitfulness that is no longer, and we mourn the fruitlessness of what has not been possible. During this phase, not only are we processing our own grief but also that of the collective. We are all inter-connected and as our intuition strengthens, we can be more aware of others' energies. Not only from other individuals but also larger groups. Our communities, country, and global energies. This can feel overwhelming. As technological information is increasingly shared, we are not only aware of our families and villages, but the whole of humanity and the planet. This can lead us to a huge sense of responsibility and disempowerment as we need to acknowledge that to some extent, we are powerless to change all things. However, we can attend to our own reality and trust that this will, in turn, bring change.

Throughout my time in the wood during my menopause, mainstream society was hit hard by the COVID-19 pandemic. In my immediate community culture, we chopped wood and carried water. We had little access to the news, other than what we were told or noticed when we took a trip into town. Unlike many, we didn't talk too much about it, sometimes this was a conscious choice as it always seemed to introduce fear, uncertainty, and anxiety and lower the vibration. At other times it was simply because it was not on the radar of our daily reality. In some ways I lived in a parallel reality. When I would speak to family or friends, they would be anxious about what they were being told regarding threats to their own health and the health of society in general. There was an enormous preoccupation with it which made it more real in their lives. The media announced huge numbers of people who were unwell or dying, which, of course, leads to mass anxiety and fear. Even though I did not hold the same perception as many in society and was not anxious about the situation, I was aware that I would experience waves of grief or fear. I knew them to not be my own, I can only imagine that I was tuning in and picking up upon the collective emotion.

For many years I heard a whisper of wanting to go into the earth, to be enveloped, held, and wrapped in her darkness. Finally, this came to be during my shamanic training whereupon we had a burial ceremony. This was a beautiful occasion; with much anticipation, nervousness, and readiness for it all. The day before the ceremony, alongside my trainee sisters and brothers, we dug our own graves together. We joked and reflected upon the earth as we dug, was it stony, hard, and unyielding or soft and easy? Did this reflect something about ourselves? This practice also gave us direct contact with the consideration and contemplation of death, not only our own but also those dear ones we had witnessed being buried. On the night of the ceremony our teachers and elders held the space by the fire, and we settled into our freshly dug graves. Wooden boards were placed across the top, followed by more soil, it was dark. A small hole was left open for air by removing a stone from the soil on top.

We told our stories, shared our tears, our challenges and achievements to our Mother, we rested in her arms, we visioned, shared our heartfelt dreams and made our prayers. We emerged from our graves with the sun rising and gave our blessings. Appreciating the sunlight and warmth of the morning, a new day and a new beginning. When I recall this ceremony, I liken it to the menopause in many ways. Including the nights by the hearth alone, with the night's blackness as company, the night listening to my sighs, cries and prayers.

During the menopause, there is often the common desire to return to the darkness. In a workshop following our discussion about the need to rest in the comfort of darkness, one woman shared that she had laid down to rest between sessions and the thought occurred to her to imagine being covered in soil, like a blanket. She rested there using her imagination to sense the comfort of being covered in earth. After a while, she got up and she said she felt refreshed and restored. This was unusual for her as she would usually tell herself, 'I've got ten minutes' and then not relax fully or deeply. So, our intention to connect with the earth and to acknowledge the healing and soothing potential of being buried, either literally or through visualisation, can be profound.

As we age and move through our middle years we are invited to contemplate and get to know death. Death begins to make itself more known. If we can let go of our fear of death, or at least lessen it, we are less resistant to ageing. We can be more accepting of change and cling less to our identity. Exploring death also supports us to acquire a different perspective on life, to evaluate what is important to us and shed any conditioned beliefs that may create an obstacle to living with more joy and depth. The menopause naturally gives us this opportunity. We are faced with our inevitable deterioration, we are invited to turn inwards to uncover and remember the old ways, the wise women ways. These are the ways of listening, of knowing how we may heal ourselves. The hag or crone comes into vision, she cuts through the illusions and petty fantasies we have held dear, she whispers the old ways and calls us to remember who we are.

During my time in the hut in the depth of the woods I was frequently visited by animal creatures, we co-existed. I was a visitor in their woodland. Over the years, many people had stayed in the hut. The birds, squirrels, mice, and rats had known where to find delicious treats, where the vulnerable spots were in the human kitchen and which cooking activities were likely to provide tasty provisions. I had a small outdoor kitchen and a metal trunk where I stored the food. Sometimes this was sufficient to maintain an easy relationship with the woodland animals but other times it was more challenging.

Once I was away for a few days, and upon my return I found that rats or squirrels had entered the hut and eaten my *tilak*. Tilak is used in Hindu and yogic traditions, applied to the eyebrow centre as a symbol of awakening *agya* chakra. The energy centre that relates to visions, intuition, and wisdom. Traditionally, menstrual blood would have been used as a sacred fluid to anoint and awaken the third eye, especially in Shakti orientated traditions. Now it is made of *kum kum* a red powder and oil, usually ghee. Rats and squirrels love oil so it was up for grabs. I had also been given some magic mushrooms (psilocybin mushrooms), which I had stored in a jar, with the lid securely closed, in the outdoor kitchen. These too had been broken into, conjuring a wonderful image of the rats and squirrels decorated with tilak and hallucinating on mushrooms! These animals were extremely dexterous, intent and focused on their desire. Often, they would wait until I left the hut and began to walk up the woodland path before they would head for the outdoor kitchen. They were like teenagers waiting for their mum to leave the house before raiding the fridge.

Interactions such as these were a reminder of how human-centric we generally are in society. Of course, sometimes it was inconvenient and a hassle to not leave a dirty plate or leftovers lying around, but overall, it was a pleasure to live alongside these woodland animals that we can learn so much from. Just prior to my decision to leave the wood in the midst of my menopause, the rats began to come into the hut at night. A couple of times running over or past my head whilst sleeping. That was a climactic point for me, a boundary had been crossed.

In spiritual circles there can be a culture of not complaining or talking too much about one's own struggles. This appears to be based on the notion of not offloading negative vibrations on others and of not reinforcing whatever's going on for you. This is based on the universal law of attraction, that wherever we put our energy, either positive or negative, it will attract more of the same. This is an important understanding to have, yet it can also produce feelings of isolation, of feeling unsupported and that one can't be authentic.

I recall trying to share how challenging this felt to me with the guardian of the land where I was living. She would say things like, 'aren't you lucky?' or 'I wonder why you are attracting that?' At the time I was having negative thoughts and feelings about being there. When living a simple life, off-grid, one's experience can oscillate from feeling incredibly blessed and unable to comprehend why everyone doesn't choose to live like this in such simple abundance, to feeling poor, wretched, marginalised, and on the fringe of society. I was attracting negative experiences that mirrored my feelings of death, decay, and depression. I became more scrupulous about leaving food crumbs around, I searched for holes to fill in the dung and mud wall plaster. Towards the end I do not know if the rats were still coming in, but I felt that they were. I experienced anxiety and hypervigilance during the night. My sleep was restless, and I would remain awake, fearful, listening sometimes into the early hours of the morning. My mind fantasised about being bitten, eaten, and attacked in my sleep. My unconscious process wrestled with feeling out of control as I moved nearer to death. This was a huge change for me as I was usually someone who would sleep easily and deeply. I experienced heart palpitations and breathing difficulties. I was experiencing the fire of *nigredo* and my container or crucible felt shaky.

It was a classic 'monster in the night' experience. It was also a classic menopausal hormone change resulting in release of cortisol, putting strain on the adrenals and nervous system akin to the fight and flight response (Rosenherg, 2017). This experience reinforced my feelings of existential loneliness and tipped into deep shame. Several months later I had the revelation that 'rats' is 'star' backwards, which put a welcomed different spin on things. There can be a deep, shameful fear that there will be no change, that we will stay here in the underworld forever void of joy, inspiration, and love. Unable to free ourselves, we will be like the walking dead, pretending to be alive when there is just empty darkness inside.

For a large period of my menopause my body felt exhausted. I could sleep for twelve hours straight, and this felt about right, but this is not so easy for most women to have. Once the adrenal glands are strained and if they are already stressed and compromised, it can be much more difficult to soothe oneself and stay in balance. I found reciting mantra during the sleepless nights helpful as it not only occupies the mind it is also soothing, helps identification with Source and keeps perspective rather than being drawn deeper into egoic fear and anxiety.

Thyroid problems are a modern-day common condition, particularly prevalent in women aged 40–50. Many of the symptoms are the same as those experienced in menopause so can go undetected (thyroiduk. org). The endocrine system is already compromised during the menopause as the ovaries slowly make less oestrogen and then eventually stop. Thyroid conditions can be amplified by adrenal stress. This means that self-care, relaxation, and resting the para-sympathetic nervous system is crucial. Practices to balance vishuddhi chakra can be helpful, as the energy centre identified with the thyroid gland. See Vishuddhi awakening practice on page 107. Herbal medicine can also help support our adrenals at these times, which is beyond the scope of this book. Support for your thyroid and to prevent imbalance include adding seaweed and brazil nuts into your diet, natural sources of iodine and selenium. There are some other books suggested in the further resources section on page 171 that can guide you as to which herbs may be helpful to you. You may also wish to consult a herbalist.

During the perimenopause phase, my body ached a lot and my bones really hurt. It's a strange sensation as we don't usually think much about our bones, especially in terms of hurting (unless broken). It was intense and as with many of these experiences no one else can see it, the pain and discomfort are not witnessed so we tend to muddle along without the care and love we need. During this time, I was connecting with my ancestors. The ancestors from my family lineage but also broader human ancestry. I had a strong impression that whatever consciousness or awareness I could muster in my own menopausal journey was as a gift and healing for the women who had come before me yet also clearing the path for the women to come. We refer to teenagers as having growing pains and this is in effect what's going on in these transition phases, the body is changing.

I began a daily practice of remembering my ancestors on my altar and spoke their names, acknowledging what they had given me and letting go of what did not serve me. This helped to give an outward expression and form to the pain. As archaeologists and scientists know, our bones carry our DNA, the genetic instructions for how we function and develop. Our bones are also our scaffolding, frame, architecture, and structure. I felt that my bones wished to realign, change and adapt. During this time, I received many downloads of information and this included the knowing that it is potentially possible to change our DNA coding and genetic imprint. It is amazing to consider that our wombs carry three generations. The eggs in our ovaries form when we are a foetus in our mother's womb and our mothers' eggs were formed in our grandmother's womb. We hold our lineage in our bodies. The healing and changes that we undertake change the unfolding of our family lineage.

I found it useful and potent to perform a ritual, collecting bone-like sticks and letting them go into a flowing stream. I honoured my ancestors by name for the gifts they have given me, but also vocalised clearly what I no longer needed to keep. Some of this was what I knew from family stories and some was unformed or unknown. In this ritual I let go and released that which prevented me from stepping into my full expression of power and creativity. There is guidance in the practice section below for you to perform a similar ritual.

Contemplation questions

🪶 How do you respond to change?

🪶 How do you feel about ageing?

🪶 How do you feel about death?

🪶 What might the gifts or teachings be from being in the Underworld?

🪶 What habits, thoughts, and beliefs no longer serve you and you wish to let go of?

🪶 Do you feel any resistance in your body and emotions about letting go?

🪶 What impressions and old stories are you still holding onto from when you were young that may be obstacles to you stepping into your sovereignty?

🪶 In which ways do you feel your ancestors have influenced your life—the gifts and the challenges? How might you release or separate from these aspects that no longer serve you?

🪶 To what extent do you feel influenced by the collective? How do you process this?

Practices to support your underworld journey

Infinite breath

As we begin to surrender and let go, we can begin to fall into a space that connects us to that which is beyond our usual sphere, that which is forever expansive and infinite.

Here are three practices that support connecting to our vibrational body, to soothe and heal. At the end of the practices make time to externalise your awareness.

Each practice can be done for 10–20 minutes or any length of time that feels right for you. They can be practised separately or as a sequence.

1) Either lie down or sit in a comfortable position in the dark or with soft candlelight. Place one hand on the heart and one hand on the womb space, bring your awareness to the natural breath.
2) Become aware of the spine from the base of the body to the crown or top of the head.
   Breathe up and down the central energy channel or *sushumna nadi*. Inhale as you imagine, sense, visualise the breath moving up this central channel and descending this channel as you exhale.
3) Visualise the infinity symbol, the figure of 8 or *lemniscate*[4] (Buxton, 2004), one orb around the womb space the other around the heart

---

[4] The lemniscate is a sacred glyph used in Lyceum tradition. It is also known as the infinity symbol in other traditions and can be used in many ways, essentially it holds the polarities that can be integrated and transcends linear time and space. See Buxton, Simon, *The Shamanic Way of the Bee* (Vermont, Destiny Books, 2004)

space. The central knot being at *manipur* chakra or the navel. Allow the breath to traverse this sacred symbol. Pause at the knot at the navel when you wish. You may wish to pause and then move your awareness in the other direction. When you are ready to complete your practice end at the central knot at manipur.

The manipur chakra or energy centre relates to our external identity, our sense of self in the world, it's our energy and 'umph'. By integrating the energies and wisdom from the womb space and heart we are drawing these qualities into an outward expression in our lives, and we can balance our energies.

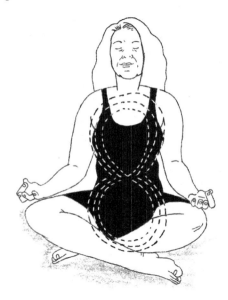

Infinite breath

Ancestral ritual

Perform a ritual to your ancestors.

Prepare the space, you may wish to light a candle.

Collect some bones or twigs that represent your ancestors.

Acknowledge what you have received from them, all that they have given you and then speak aloud your paternal and maternal lineage or family names as far back as you know.

With clear intention let go of any patterns or beliefs that you are carrying that no longer serve you. Release these patterns by letting go of the bones or twigs into a fire, place of water, or other natural place of your choosing.

Dark goddess sacred fire

Traditionally a yogic fire would be held in a copper pyramid or *kund*. You can adapt and use a fire outside, an open fire or wood burner. The intention is the most important ingredient.

Daniel Odier in *Tantric Kali* (Odier, 2016) outlines that auspicious times to worship Kali are on the dark moon, on Tuesdays and at dusk or darkness. Perform the sacred fire at a time that feels right for you.

You may use a real fire or imaginary one.

If using an imaginary fire prepare as you would for meditation. Imagine in front of you a red triangle, the point or apex towards you. In the centre imagine a burning fire.

If using a manifest fire—gather what you need: wood, some water, petals, or any other offerings you would like to make. Traditionally this would be *samagri*, a blend of herbs, petals, and incense. You may like to make an indigenous samagri using sacred herbs native to where you live and dry them before blending and using on your sacred fire. Rosemary, sage, chamomile, hawthorn berries and leaves, rose petals, apple blossom, honey, propolis, and tree resin all make lovely offerings. You will need some oil, traditionally *ghee* or clarified butter but olive oil can also be used. This oil is a lubricant to the fire.

Decide on how many times you wish to repeat the mantra. One-hundred and eight times or any division of that number (fifty-four, twenty-seven) is traditional in yoga. You may wish to use a *mala* (string of beads) to count.

Repeating the name of the Goddess is powerful because it contains and is an expression of the vibration of that deity. It also stills the mind which allows us to connect with our own higher self. In this practice we are offering our practice to the dark and wild Goddess Kali. If you prefer you can focus on any other Goddess of your choosing.

Kali mantra:

Om krim Kaliyai namaha

(Phonetic pronunciation- aum kreem kali-i nama-ha)

Place any offerings into the fire as you repeat the mantra.

If you are using your imagination to create a fire, then imagine making your offerings as you repeat the mantra.

As you perform this practice know that you are honouring the dark Goddess as you, that you are honouring the darkness in all her aspects, the unconscious, the shadow, the hidden.

By bringing the light of awareness to these shadow aspects we can help these unrecognised parts to flow and can assimilate them.

When finished sit by the fire and absorb the energies from the practice. Express gratitude if you wish and conclude the practice.

Meditation—healing and integrating the womb's stories

Sitting or lying down in *shavasana*[5] or semi-supine position, with the knees bent and resting one against the other. Allow the body to settle and become still.

Become aware of the natural breath.

Imagine, sense, or visualise a light at agya chakra. You can focus on the eyebrow centre and then move inwards allowing the awareness to rest at the centre of the head.

With each inhalation imagine the light becoming brighter, it may also change shape, be static or move. Just allow whatever occurs naturally to be.

Inhale and exhale into agya chakra.

After several minutes allow your attention to move down to the heart space, the front of the body at the centre of the chest between your breasts.

Imagine, sense, or visualise this light at the heart centre or anahat chakra, breathing in and out of this energy centre, allowing the light to become brighter with every breath.

Then descending down the central pathway (*sushumna nadi*) to the womb space.

Once more imagine this light in this space and gently, gradually begin to move this light as a wand or eraser, moving it around your yoni and womb, around the ovaries, cervix, fallopian tubes, vagina, vaginal lips,

---

[5] *Shavasana* or *corpse* pose is an excellent resting pose and I refer to it several times during the book. Lie on your back, allow a space between the ankles, arms by side of body, a space between the arms and the side of body. A still symmetrical body. Allow the weight of the body to release into the earth.

bringing healing to all areas where you feel drawn to bring this light. There may be a feeling of stuck energy, blockage or shadow. Gently, use the light to soften and transform these areas of trapped energy.

As you heal and give loving care to yourself, you could also acknowledge all the experiences that your yoni has had; this may include giving birth, miscarriage, abortion, sex enjoyed, sex unwanted, guilty sex, sexual trauma, shame, and pleasure.

Take your time, you may wish to repeat this practice daily for several days, allowing whatever arises to be.

You may use the light without having any association or story and that is fine; as always, follow your intuition. Allow time and space for assimilation.

Burial meditation

You may wish to record yourself reading this script aloud so you can play it back to yourself and deeply relax.

Lie in shavasana or semi-supine position.

Feel yourself supported by the earth. Bring your awareness to all the parts of the body in contact with the ground.

With every breath allow yourself to release a little more. The body is heavy and relaxed. No doing, just being.

Imagine yourself in nature, perhaps a favourite spot you know.

Imagine, sense, or visualise layers of earth covering you, it may be as thick or as thin as you are comfortable with. Allow yourself to relax and surrender, letting go of any resistance.

Relax deeply. Imagine that any holding, whether physical, mental or emotional is being absorbed by the earth. With every exhalation allow yourself to let go a little more, relaxing and surrendering deeply to Mother Earth.

Alternatively, in a private place in nature, lie down and cover yourself with soil or leaves. Follow the meditation guidance above.

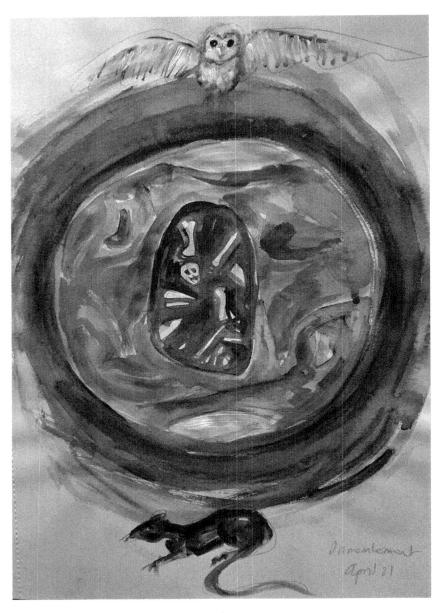

Dismemberment

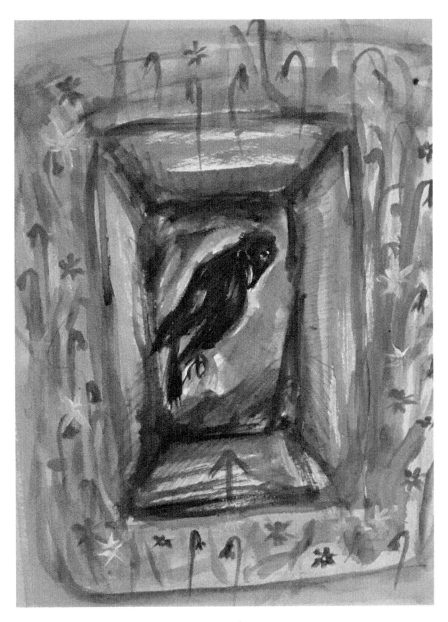

Burial

CHAPTER 4

Who's in your Circle?

During the menopause nothing feels quite right. The people that we thought we loved, the friends that always 'got us' suddenly don't or we may be irritated or feel like we are playing a role and we are unable to be authentic with them anymore. When we change, one of the hardest things can be when people around us unconsciously want us to stay the same. It's a neat fit and has worked well, why change it? When we meet them, it can be very difficult not to slip back into old ways; it's a gentle, unconscious coercion to stay the same, to respond in the way we always have. We are expected to exhibit the same energetic frequency, to be the same person they think they know and love and to continue on with the habitual dynamic of relating. However, there is only so much of this that we can tolerate, and inevitably, if you are being true to yourself and the people around you, you will change. Friendships will begin to fade, perhaps relationships will end. This can be a time of feeling alienated and alone, which can be painful. Of course, it's ironic because part of you craves to be alone. If you have a partner and family, you can still experience this isolation. Ultimately, as with any significant event, we walk alone in our existential unfolding.

One of the reasons a period of retreat is so valuable during this time is because it can allow you to get comfortable with the changes you are undertaking for yourself, before taking yourself back out into the world. Family and old friends may energetically lean on you to be your good old self. As you settle into and firm up your new identity you are more able to navigate these subtle and sometimes not so subtle interactions. You are more able to maintain your boundaries. The new 'you' can be like a spring seedling, still emerging, still needing protection from the different external conditions. This is discussed in more detail in Chapter 6, 'New Threads Stitched Over Old'.

It can feel that our human allies fall away or don't show up in the way they used to. However, this does not mean you are doing it alone. A beautiful way of supporting yourself can be to create a circle of allies. This means calling in and visualising who is in your circle. It's a bit like that game of, 'Who would you invite to your perfect dinner party?'. Ancestors, role models, dear friends, teachers, light beings and animal guides. So, who do you want to invite to be in your circle? The circle should include only those beings that you feel totally supported by, where there is ease, harmony, and acceptance.

This circle can be drawn upon whenever needed. It may be that you choose as a daily practice to sit quietly and imagine being with them, even perhaps listen to what they wish to offer in support of your journey. I recall chuckling to myself as I would be surprised at how many amazing beings I had in my circle; I felt elated, blessed, supported, and grateful. On one dimension I might have felt alone but on another I was far from being alone and isolated. They may include an animal, a spiritual teacher, a spiritual being, a human who is alive or dead that feels solid and supportive, not restricting your expansion with expectation and assumptions.

One of my main allies during this time and ongoing is Goddess Kali. She is the ultimate Mother as she transcends time and space and embodies the cycle of birth and death. She is the One who fiercely loves. At this time, she is an amazing ally to foster and I related to her enormously. The wildness, the intensity, the acceptance of all. Devotion to Kali is intense, some would avoid it. But if you are a conscious seeker on your menopause journey, merging yourself in this rite of passage and not wanting to avoid or hide, then who could be a better companion?

I found repetition of the mantra extremely helpful, not only in giving the mind something to focus on but also to align with Her. I had a statue of her on my altar, and on dark moon nights or at other times, if I felt inspired, I would chant to her and make offerings. I would delight in performing the practice of *abhieshek*. This is a Hindu ritual where sacred substances are poured over a statue of a deity whilst chanting mantra. This was traditionally reserved for male Brahmins (Hindu priests) so what a joy to shatter this taboo in the way that Kali would love and do it my way when I wished. Kali calls for respect, love and devotion and by performing these rituals we can channel these feelings. Over her statue I would lovingly pour honey, ghee, spring water, rice, blood (if I could get it), and sing to Her. The more you give to her or any deity the more alive and deeper the relationship becomes. It's like anything, the more we can give the more we will receive.

Kali gives us permission to reside in the darkness, at the crossroads, to allow being in between, to surf neither one thing or the other, the betwixt, non-linear, and unfathomable. After a while I did feel that I needed a break from her fierce love, to soften the penetration and intensity. I began to chant Goddess Lakshmi mantra and chants. Lakshmi is associated with good fortune and sweetness, and we will explore Her further in Chapter 8, 'Weaving the Golden Thread.' This is the beauty of the myriad of Goddesses and Gods, whether yogic, Celtic or other, that we can choose and resonate with different aspects and qualities at different times. Spirit, Source, Shakti or Consciousness reveals itself to us in numerous ways for our benefit. Energy takes shape and manifests in many ways to help support us on our human journey.

Another major ally during menopause is darkness. Society teaches us that darkness is negative and bad. We have gone to great lengths to eliminate or reduce darkness from our lives with electricity, including streetlights, and security lights. However, in many esoteric traditions it is recognised that the darkness can lead us to inner light and illumination. The deeper we can allow ourselves to fall, the higher we can climb, as the old adage states, 'as above, so below'. The deeper we can feel our wounds and the extremes of our human pain and vulnerability, the greater our potential for expansion and for filling the heart with light. Don't get me wrong, I'm not saying that we need to suffer but I am saying that if we can allow ourselves to meet ourselves where we are honestly, that this can be incredibly liberating. Society's attempt to get rid of darkness is an expression of avoidance and resistance to exploring our unconscious. There is a projection of fear and danger onto others and this is continually reinforced.

Darkness can be experienced as restful, soft, and velvety in texture, it can soothe us into deep rest. I have increasingly found bright lights challenging and almost painful at times. There are several ways to contemplate this light sensitivity. The pituitary gland is part of the endocrine system, linked to agya chakra, and, as our wise woman is activated, it can lead us to spiritual expansion. It likes the dark. We have grown up in a culture that values light; we are surrounded by electricity, as soon as dusk comes, if not before, people turn on their lights. Car lights come on at the slightest dip in light. We miss the beauty of dusk, that in between time where the veil between the manifest world and spiritual world is thinnest. We are taught that darkness needs to be avoided. In the same vein our own shadowy realms are also avoided.

Down in the wood, the guardian of the land would discourage the use of torches, saying that light was an insult to the darkness. I generally have poor night vision and did surreptitiously use my torch down the winding path to my hut. Apparently, previous tenants who were torchless sometimes never found their way home and slept on the path until dawn. It is an interesting thought about how we intrude upon the darkness with light, does darkness intrude upon light in the same way? Symbolically, we play with the notions of what we wish to see or keep in the dark. Ann Mankowitz (1984) describes the conflict between the need to know and the fear of knowing. During menopause we are faced with bringing into sight, vison, or light what may have been previously avoided, denied, and feared. This takes courage and calls upon the spiritual warrior within us.

The other key ally for us is nature. Being in nature is inherently healing. The patterns of nature remind us on subtle levels of our own connection with nature. The elements reflect to us what we are made of. During one retreat I spent a full day exploring each element in turn. This was a beautiful practice as it allowed me time to explore and appreciate each element and reflect upon how it is in my own being and my relationship to it.

Earth is connected to our solidity, our roots, how secure we feel, a sense of home. It is our flesh and bones, matter turning eventually to compost. It is the most static of the elements, it can bring stability and permanence. Consider if you feel a security and trust in life and in your foundations.

The element of water is *apas* in Sanskrit, which means to pervade. It offers us emotions, fluidity, our capacity to move and flow with change and circumstance. It can be still warm waters or fast flowing rivers or expansive oceans. There is an impermanence attributed to its altering state. It is our blood, bile, and tears. We are vastly made up of water. Masaru Emoto's (2005) experiments revealed how water has a vibrational energy by exposing water to various words, pictures or music, then freezing the water. When he examined the frozen crystals, they revealed pristine mandala-like crystals of the water received affirming positive words and distorted, irregular shapes if they received negative input. This illustrates how the vibrations that surround us can have profound impact on our health. Consider your relationship to water and the flow of life.

Fire is the spark, the warmth of the hearth, energy, the electricity between synapses, the impulse to act and provides light. It ignites our passions and desires. It is action and can destroy impurities. Are you quick to temper, reactive, irritable? Agni or fire is also known as *tejas*, to sharpen. Fire consumes and transforms matter, which is why it is important in our initiation process. It can cause instability and in the tantric practice of Tattwa Shuddhi[6] is linked to the area between the heart and navel, responsible for digestion. As the element of fire is often heightened in our system during menopause it is interesting in relation to heart palpitations and irregular sensations often experienced during this phase.

The element of air is linked to movement and thoughts. It is the wind moving the clouds, seeds, and pollen. Air is in a gaseous form and not physically visible. It is energy in motion and can create instability. We can feel the winds of change. Take some time to connect with this element and feel into it. The pleasurable sensation of a cool breeze on hot skin or the exhilaration of a wild wind around your house on a stormy day. Too much air can make us feel ungrounded, flighty, and erratic. Air is our breath that connects us from the inside to the outside, a thread tethering us to everything.

Ether is often joined with the element air because of its subtle nature, but their differentiation is important. Ether is the space in between, the lightness in the space between matter and molecules. It is the feeling of expansion, and spaciousness that extends beyond the human limitations that we can touch upon. It is the space between our organs and

---

[6] Tattwa shuddhi is a tantric practice that purifies and transforms the body, from the most subtle to the physical levels.

cells, it is the space between our inhalation and exhalation. Ether is the space between ourselves and our not-self.

All the elements are expressions of Source and in all things. We are made from the elements, so when we consider and reflect on how we resonate with each element it can be revealing and can support us in making shifts in how to realign with aspects of ourselves. As we reflect on the interplay of elements and how they express themselves within us, with greater awareness, we can make amendments through breath, action, conscious thought and diet to bring balance and equilibrium. When we are aware of the element expressing dominantly through us at any given time we can adjust and adapt to bring increased harmony to our system. For example, if I have been on the computer a while, I may notice that my thoughts are more rapid and unsettled, an expression of increased vata and the element of air. I could then decide to connect to the earth element to become more grounded and *sattvic* through walking outside barefoot for ten minutes. If I am feeling irritable and can feel my fire flaring up, I can drink some cooling hibiscus tea, do some slow movement or a moon meditation to increase connection with the water element to balance the heat I am experiencing.

Contemplation questions

To what extent do you feel supported in your life?

Can you gain greater clarity about what support you need and who (other than yourself) can offer it?

Are there relationships in your life that you no longer resonate with?

What is your relationship with nature?

What is your relationship with the elements of earth, water, fire, air, and ether?

Are you able to ask for help? If this is not easy for you reflect upon this resistance and the emotions and thoughts around this.

How do you feel about inviting forth a circle of allies?

Practices to support you in feeling supported

Yoga nidra—exploring the elements

Yoga nidra is a deep relaxation that is translated as *yogic sleep*. It is an excellent practice to assimilate changes, to balance and calm the nervous system and restore the mind and body, especially if you are having disrupted sleep.

For this practice, I suggest you read aloud the script and record it so you can use it when you wish. Read it in a clear voice at a steady pace.

Ensure that you won't be interrupted.

(Begin) Lie in shavasana or semi-supine position. Allow a little space between your arms and the side of your body and space between the ankles. You may like to place a bolster or folded blanket beneath your knees or lower thighs.

Remove any bulky jewellery or glasses.

During the practice, I will refer to your *sankalpa*. A sankalpa is your resolve and intention, it is a short positive statement about your life that you will repeat several times during the practice. The seed of the sankalpa is planted in your unconscious, allowing it to flourish without resistance. Choose something that has real value and meaning to you before you begin the practice. A sankalpa is an affirming statement spoken in the present tense, for example, 'I am moving towards fulfilling my soul's purpose.'

Set an intention to remain awake and aware during the practice.

Make any final adjustments to body or clothing. Allow the body to become still, only move if there is pain or significant discomfort.

Become aware of the connection between body and ground. All the parts of the body in connection with the body and ground. The feet, legs, buttocks, back, all the parts of the back, hands and arms, and the back of the head.

With every breath allow the body to become more relaxed and have a sense of letting go into the earth, knowing that She is supporting you and there is nothing for you to do but listen to the instructions.

Silently repeat your sankalpa, the positive affirming statement about your life. Repeat it with deep faith and conviction.

The next part of the practice is the rotation of awareness around the body. Follow the voice and as each part of the body is named, bring your awareness to that body part and mentally repeat the name of that part of the body.

Awareness to right hand ... right hand thumb ... second finger ... third finger ... fourth finger ... fifth finger ... palm of hand ... back of hand ... wrist ... forearm ... elbow ... upper arm ... right shoulder ... armpit ... side of body ... waist ... hip ... thigh ... knee ... back of knee ... shin ... calf ... heel ... top of right foot ... sole of foot ... big toe ... second toe ... third toe ... fourth toe ... fifth toe ...

Awareness now to left hand ... left hand thumb ... second finger ... third finger ... fourth finger ... fifth finger ... palm of hand ... back of hand ... wrist ... forearm ... elbow ... upper arm ... left shoulder ... armpit ... side of body ... waist ... hip ... thigh ... knee ... back of knee ... shin ... calf ... heel ... top of left foot ... sole of foot ... big toe ... second toe ... third toe ... fourth toe ... fifth toe ...

Awareness to right buttock ... left buttock ... lower back ... middle back ... upper back ... the whole of the back ... the spinal column ... the whole of the back ... back of neck ... back of head ... top of head ... forehead ... right temple ... left temple ... right ear ... left ear ... right eyebrow ... left eyebrow ... the space between the eyebrows ... right eye ... left eye ... right cheek ... left cheek ... right nostril ... left nostril ... tip of nose ... upper lip ... lower lip ... space where lips meet ... tongue ... teeth ... chin ... jaw ... throat ... right collar bone ... left collar bone ... right breast ... left breast ... centre of the chest ... upper abdomen ... lower abdomen ... navel ... the womb space ... the elimination organs ...

The whole of the right side of body ... whole of left side of body ... right and left side of body together ... the front of body ... back of body ... front and back of the body together ...the whole of the body ... awareness of the whole of the body, whole body awareness.

Become aware now of your breath ... the body breathing in and body breathing out ... feel the sensation of breath on your nostrils, sensation of breath ... in the upper lungs ... lower lungs ... abdomen ... awareness of abdomen expanding with the inhalation and contracting with exhalation ... become aware of the body breathing ... continue being aware of the natural breath for three minutes.

Allow yourself to experience the sensation of coolness in the body ... the whole body feeling colder and colder ... imagine you are walking outside on a cold winter's day ... you are wearing no coat or shoes ... the cold from the ground is rising up through the body ... the sensation of coldness in the feet in the toes … fingers …. and hands … the arms and legs, so cold you could shiver … a cold body … the whole torso, head and skull feeling so, so cold. Allow yourself to fully experience the sensation of a cold body. Release the sensation of coldness in the body now … fully let go of the sensation of a coldness in the body.

Become aware of the sensation of heat in the body … allow the body to feel warmer and warmer. Surrender the whole body to the sensation of heat … it's as if you're walking on a hot summer's day and the sun is beating down on you … imagine walking on hot sand … feel the sensation of heat in the feet … rising up into the legs … hips … back … arms … and hands … the whole torso feeling so, so hot … the head, and skull so hot … you are so hot you could perspire … the whole body feeling warmer and warmer … the skin absorbing the heat into every pore and cell of the body … fully allow yourself to experience the sensation of heat … release the sensation of heat in the body now … fully let go of the sensation of a heat in the body.

Bring your awareness to your eyebrow centre, the activation point for agya chakra … allow yourself to breath here … inhale into eyebrow centre … exhale from eyebrow centre … continue this for several breaths.

Become aware of the body boundary … the skin boundary and the space inside … become aware of the organs in the body … and the space between the organs … the spaces between the bones … become aware of the element of ether within the body … become aware of movement in the body … the natural breath … the element of air … become aware of heat in the body … the process of digestion in the body … the temperature of the body … awareness of the element of fire in the body … bring your awareness of bodily fluids … the blood and lymph circulating … saliva in the mouth … become aware of the element of water in the body … become aware of the density of the body … the bones and skeleton … and muscles … the solidity of muscles ….awareness of the earth element within the body … bring your awareness to the whole body … expanding as it inhales … gently contracting with the exhalation for three minutes.

Let go of awareness of the elements within the body now … bring the awareness to the heart space … It is time for you to repeat your sankalpa once again, repeating it several times to yourself with faith and conviction that it is manifesting in your life. Release your sankalpa now … become aware of your whole body, the outline and physicality of your body … know that the yoga nidra will soon be coming to an end … become aware of the contact between floor and feet … legs … contact between the back and the ground … the ground making contact with the arms and hands … and the back of the head … all the points of contact between body and ground … become aware of the room that you are in … noticing the body breathing and allow a couple of deeper breaths … now that the yoga nidra is concluding … continue to externalise your awareness … gently allow the head to roll to one side then the other … bring gentle movement to fingers and toes … bring the knees up to the chest and give yourself a hug … stretch and yawn … when you are ready you can sit up … take your time.

Meditation—circle of support

Come to a comfortable seated position or lie in shavasana or semi-supine.

Allow the body to come to stillness and become aware of the breath.

Call forth your chosen circle, see or sense your circle taking their places around you or next to you.

Request a healing that you need at this time or ask a question to help guide you.

Allow the answer to come in any form it needs to, you may hear, see, sense it or nature may bring it forward. Be open with all your senses to receive.

Express your appreciation before closing the circle.

Creating a sacred bundle[7]

Set aside some undisturbed time in nature.

Set your intention to find objects from nature that represent each member of your circle; for example, if I have a particular animal or teacher that I resonate with I will ask internally or aloud for a natural object to offer itself as that animal to join my bundle.

---

[7] Creating a sacred bundle is common in many shamanic traditions, including core shamanism as taught by the Sacred Trust and the Lyceum. It is a way to bridge the Spirit or non-ordinary reality with the ordinary manifest world.

Without relying on your cognitive mind, wait and feel to see what shows up, often the perfect piece of wood will pretty much leap into your hand.

When you have collected your circle, tie it in ribbon, cloth, string or twine made from any natural materials such as hemp or stinging nettles. You may like to anoint this in some way. You can use body fluids such as sweat, urine and blood.

You may wish to keep your bundle with you, attaching it to your body for a time or placing it on your altar to offer power and support.

When the time feels right, which may be in weeks, months or years, you can let it go with gratitude. Returning it to nature, to the earth, into the fire or any place of water. Your sacred bundle may also be with you during your wise woman celebration, see Chapter 9, 'Wise Woman Celebration'.

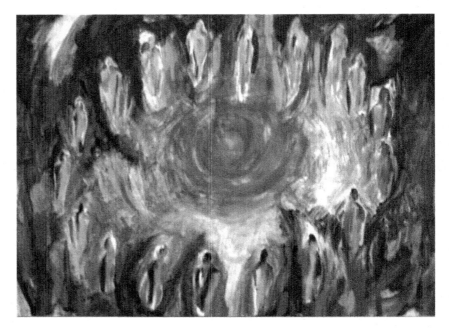

Circle of Support

CHAPTER 5

Chiron's in the House

For those of you who have an interest in astrology, you will know that this time in our lives also corresponds with the significant astrological phase called the *Chiron Return*. I am no professional astrologer, but I have developed an interest in it. I appreciate that this corresponds with the menopause so perfectly; it can help when the universe shows us something that helps put context to our own experience.

Chiron is a constellation and the wounded healer. Between the age of forty-nine and fifty-one we enter our Chiron Return. Perfect; this is what is commonly known as the midlife crisis. It's where we are tempted to leave the kids, take a younger lover, and flee to the hills. It is a potent time where there is the potential to turn old core wounds into gifts. During the menopause it can be hard to see that one may have any gifts or do anything with them, even if they were found. This relates to the intensity of feelings that we can experience.

Our Chiron Return prompts us to consider, 'What am I going to do with the last part of my life?'. In her book 'Chiron and the Healing Journey' Roselyn Reinhart (Reinhart, 1989) writes:

"… sickness, depression and inner confrontation with the self may occur; this time its purpose is the integration of the entire life cycle thus far, an inner reviewing and restructuring …"

As we explored in Chapter 3, 'The Underworld', the transition stage of initiation is where past trauma and wounds rise to consciousness. Like a pond where the murk has laid on the bottom, the dark Goddess gives it a stir and there it is, visible and tangible. We all carry these wounds whether it is deep seated imprints of abandonment, rejection, exploitation, a feeling of unworthiness or isolation. Facing these wounds appears to be an essential part of the menopause initiation.

If you have your personal astrological chart created you can see where your Chiron is placed, each house having a particular emphasis in your life. Reinhart gives a detailed account of this process. In the Greek myth Chiron faces exile and rejection from his mother causing a deep wound. Reinhart describes that Chiron was tutored by Apollo who is linked to divination and prophecy and Artemis, Apollo's brother, who presided over wild places, women's rites of passage and plant medicine. So, as we begin to explore this myth we can feel how poignant it is for the menopausal women as she grows into her wise woman.

Chiron is wounded by being struck by an arrow in the leg. In his suffering he searches for relief and healing. Ring any bells? Chiron's perseverance seemed to pay off as his wound was healed through an exchange with Prometheus. Interestingly, the constellation that is Chiron, 'Centaurus' is used for navigation and finding our way (Reinhart, 1989).

In this story we see soul expansion and growth, the transformation of a wound to a gift. Another star was discovered, known as Chaiklo, the wife of Chiron (Reinhart, 1989). This star is associated with the feminine and the heart chakra, it is also related to the balance and harmony between the feminine and masculine. She speaks to our capacity to heal others and ourselves. The couple point towards how we can support the healing of the sacred feminine and sacred masculine, a theme that we explore further in Chapter 7, 'The Priestess is in the Temple'. The centaur is often depicted as masculine and yet this half human, half horse also relates to the feminine.

In a non-ordinary journey, I journeyed to the Spirit of a nearby sacred mountain.

I saw a bowl of light as I approached. The guardians asked, 'anything to declare?' I replied that I had egoic pride and insecurities. As I spoke my energy field became brighter and stronger. I went to the water spring at the foot of the mountain and saw a serpent. I followed the serpent and descended down into a dark chamber and tunnel. There were other animals with me guiding me. I saw a huge column of light and a centaur emerged, I see that I am a centaur too and we walk together over the mountain. We stand together, head to tail, tail to head, as if one huge horse, the lemniscate moving between and around our hearts, connected us as one heart.

This journey revealed not only the descent into the underworld but also the light that came from that descent. The journey was also supported by other Beings. The serpent, an animal guide that is linked to kundalini energy and spiritual awakening was at the spring, a symbol of new beginnings, refreshment and purity. The union with the male centaur brought the healing and integration of the feminine and masculine aspects, leading to one huge heart.

As half human and half horse, Chiron is a mythological figure that we can easily relate to as we integrate our physical body with our energy body. It also links to the duality and polarity of our experience as explored in Chapter 7. I have met many women who resonate with Beings or mythological creatures who combine two aspects. Often, we feel that we are not one thing or another, but both. Like the centaur, the *mermaid* and *selkie* are Beings who we can easily resonate with during our transformation (Blakie, 2019). They exist in the betwixt and between realms. These magical figures who are half human, half fish or seal are neither of the sea or land. During our initiation we can identify with the feeling that we do not belong fully to one place nor the other. These Beings inhabit the places, the bridge, where metamorphosis unfolds. We resonate with shapeshifting, adapting, and flowing, our capacity to be present as human and spirit, of valuing our freedom and independence. These are aspects that the Chiron Return points us to.

As we move through the menopause initiation we shift our primary awareness in life to spiritual expansion, this being the return phase. From the perspective of the chakras, we are moving from perceiving and experiencing the world from the lower three energy centres to orientating primarily from the upper chakras and the heart chakra. This shift is challenging as we wish to relate from the heart space, from a place of love, compassion, and acceptance and yet we are habitually pro-grammed to relate from a place of security, power, and self-gratification. Brofman (2003) acknowledges this as an evolutionary transition, which resonates well with my own experience and that of other women. We have a foot in both realities so to speak. Like Chiron and the mermaid, we are experiencing and expressing both aspects in our lives.

This transition from where we live our lives from also relates to physical sensations and experiences during menopause. Heart palpita-tions and anxiety can be usefully perceived from this philosophy, as the physical body aligns with our evolution into lighter, more refined energy frequencies. This is where energetic healing such as the use of sound can be helpful in supporting our integration.

Part of our menopausal journey is to look in the mirror with honesty. Until now you may not have explored certain aspects of yourself. Some-times psychotherapy can offer a space for us to explore our perceptions and ways of relating to ourselves and others which can be helpful. It can help shine a light upon the dynamics that we have been living by which had seemed the norm to us, only to realise often that they are not the norm but dysfunctional or even abusive. One of the processes of this initiation can be that we come to a place of accepting the idiosyn-crasies of our personality. We come to know our trigger points well, to the extent that we are more able to laugh at them and have more com-passion for the wounds we carry. It is not necessarily about getting rid of these familiar wounds but holding them in a new or different way.

Psychotherapy can, however, also potentially keep us within a place of identifying with an old aspect of ourselves. If we are continu-ally repeating an old story, it can reinforce it rather than diminish and resolve it. This is where our wise woman can step forward and use dis-cernment to know when we need which medicine: whether to explore our past to help resolve experiences and relationships, to focus on the here and now or to intentionally create the path before us. The meno-pausal journey usually requires us to move between all of these places. Reinhart (1989) likens the process of digesting our past sufficiently to create compost with which to nourish the next phase of our life.

Often, we have been taught to look outside ourselves for the answers, to go to a doctor, therapist, or healer but we are increasingly called to turn within and consult our inner Guru or wise woman for the guid-ance that we need. This is like a muscle that needs to be developed and refined. Such explorations can support us in finding insights towards our own healing and our role as a healer. For example, if our wound was that we were restricted to communicate genuinely with others, our relief from that wound and our gift to others may be to enable others to find their voice authentically.

As we have previously explored, this is a time where we are drawn inwards and need solitude. Our capacity to continue social interaction as expected can be compromised. This is also a time when our experiences of trauma can rise to the surface. As with the Chiron Return, I was inspired to see that the explorations of the nervous system, particularly the work of Stanley Rosenberg (2017) also relate neatly to the menopause experience.

When we are healthy and in balance, in response to external experiences, we can move from being relaxed to alarmed and back again as needed. However, what can happen is that we can become stuck in a fight-or-flight response. The nervous system regulates organ functioning and many common problems, many of which are commonly experienced during menopause. These are related to automatic nervous system dysfunction. The vagal nerve is one of the cranial nerves and Rosenberg is one of an increasing number of health practitioners to highlight the importance of restoring healthy functioning. For many of us it can be part of our healing process to explore and process trauma and working with the vagal nerve can be one helpful avenue.

This is also a time where Goddess Durga can support us. Goddess Durga is the warrior. She has courage and is one-pointed in her focus. In the scriptures of yoga and tantra she overcomes demons in her battle to protect the world. These demons can be seen as a metaphor for overcoming our inner demons, or unhelpful egoic aspects, as we move through our transformation. She is depicted as having eight arms and in each of these arms she holds a weapon. She rides a tiger or lion and wears a red sari and gold crown. She 'kicks arse' when needed, she is unconcerned with placating and compromising, being obsequious or submissive. She speaks her truth and stands in her power without apology. She protects and can bring about revolution. She unleashes spiritual transformation in the form of Shakti moving within our innermost Being. Durga invites us to step up and stand in our own power. It is helpful to remind yourself about the battles you wish to fight and those you can leave be and the protection you and yours need.

During our menopause Durga can be a powerful ally as she can give us the courage and stamina to persevere and know we can overcome the challenges that we face. As we face our core wounds and aspects of our personality that need to be transmuted, invoking Goddess Durga can feel supportive. We can invoke her through meditation, prayer, mantra, and chanting. As with many of the other practices our intention is fundamental. As described previously, we can also offer our devotion and gratitude.

Contemplation questions

🖋 What do you regard as your core wounds?

🖋 If you have someone that knows you intimately ask them what they regard as your core wounds and see what they say.

🖋 How might these wounds be healed?

🖋 How might these wounds become healing for others?

🖋 What might you need from outside yourself (if anything) to facilitate more understanding about your wounds?

🖋 When you consider the transformation of these wounds into treasure what response do you have?

🖋 Which mythological being do you relate to? Explore why you relate to them. You may find it useful to use art making, body, and voice work.

Practices to ride your Chiron return

Journal

Journal freely and spontaneously about your core wounds, take care not to blame others for these wounds. It is more about seeing them from an eagle's perspective.

Rewrite what you have written but this time change the wording to include the transmutation. Even if you are not feeling it yet, play with it, see if it is possible to align with that new vibration and feel into what it feels like.

For example, rather than 'I carry the wounds of being too serious and feeling unsafe to have fun' to 'my gifts and healing to others is that I can facilitate others connecting with their inner child, allowing them to feel safe to have fun and experience joy' or 'My core wound is that I don't trust others' to 'I am learning to trust the universe, so I can relax in the presence of others, knowing that everything is ok.'

Wound healing meditation

Sit in a comfortable position.

Allow the spine to lift and a sense of grounding down toward the earth through your sitting bones.

Become aware of the skin boundary to your body. Draw your attention to this body boundary.

Begin to tune into seeing with your non-corporeal vision. Where, if anywhere, might your core wound or wounds be held in the body. For example, there may be a feeling or knowing that a stagnant energy in the hip or a longstanding discomfort in the abdomen is a physical manifestation of this wound you carry.

Allow your awareness to rest here, cultivate the attitude of care and compassion. If the mind wanders just gently bring it back to this area.

As you become aware of your natural breath, imagine or sense that you are inhaling healing light into the body and with intention allow that healing breath to fill the area on the exhalation. You may like to imagine this breath as a colour or see it as a vibration.

When ready, release the practice and externalise your awareness.

Shapeshift

Do this practice when you are feeling grounded and emotionally robust, as you are moving into and then back out of non-ordinary consciousness. You may like to ask a friend to hold the space for you.

Set your intention to explore, experience, and to connect with an animal.

In a safe space explore and play with sound and movement. This may include discordant music or a shamanic drumbeat (you may wish to use a recording of a shamanic journey beat).

Allow your body to move you beyond your mind's control. The Lyceum refer to this as the *theatre of ambiguous behaviour*, which is another way of shifting awareness to 'deliberately undertake actions and thoughts that are doubtful in meaning to yourself' (Buxton, 2004). Perhaps there is an animal that you would like to connect with, whether mythological or in this reality. As you move and sound begin to invite that Being into your own energy field.

Naturally allow this to unfold and if it feels right to you, begin to merge and change into this Being. Feel the difference in breathing, body structure, senses, and movement. Continue for a time in this way.

After a while, perhaps 10–20 minutes, allow the drumbeat (or another method), to bring yourself back into focus and ordinary awareness.

Give thanks to the Being who you have explored with. Release them fully and allow more of your own identity to expand and fill out.

Welcome yourself back. Say your name out loud and externalise your awareness. Connect to the earth and your breath. Familiarise yourself with your usual activities and persona.

Be aware of the effects of the shapeshifting. Take your time and, when ready, journal your experience.

Invoking Goddess Durga

Sit in a comfortable position.

Allow the spine to lift and a sense of grounding down toward the earth through your sitting bones.

Become aware of your natural breath, the body inhaling and the body exhaling.

Bring to mind the image of Goddess Durga—riding a tiger, wearing red, a gold crown, and her jewels, her eight arms brandishing weapons. As you visualise her, begin to feel her qualities of strength, courage and determination.

Hold in mind the qualities that you would like to develop at this time, perhaps the courage to speak your truth or to let go of an old wound or story line and ask for what you need.

Repeat the mantra *OM DUM DURGAYAI NAMAHA*
(phonetic pronunciation: *aum doom door gah yi nuh muh hu*)
Salutations to Goddess Durga who overcomes all obstacles.

Synchronise your breath with the mantra.

If you prefer, you can call to her in your own language, for example:
"Oh Goddess Durga, I honour you as Shakti the Supreme Mother. I ask for your help that I may walk my path with courage and speak my truth. Blessing to you dear One."

Continue focusing on breath and mantra for as long as you feel comfortable to do so, 10–30 minutes is a nice length of time.

Gradually, release the mantra and the visualisation.

Become aware of your body in contact with the ground once more and take time to externalise your awareness before completing your practice.

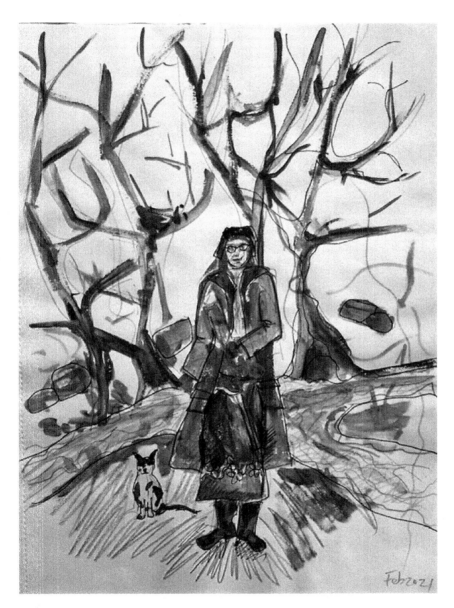

Courage of Goddess Durga (*Prepared for battle
with feline guide and helper*)

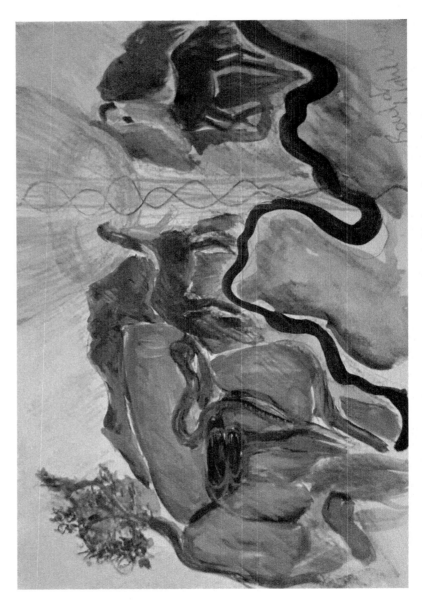

Centaurs (Centaurs meet at the bowl of light at the Mountain)

CHAPTER 6

New Threads Woven Over Old

As we move through the underworld or transition initiation phase something begins to stir. After the intensity of that peak time, we begin to feel the first sign of emergence as we slowly make our ascent. There are signs of moving from an internal focus to a more outward perspective. We are not yet ready to integrate fully back into our community and return, but we begin to feel the gentle ripples of inspiration giving seeds of hope and renewed energy. Here we meet the *albedo* alchemical stage. Our tears and sweat have offered liquid to the ashes of what remains of our previous sense of self. Our sweat and tears bind our grief and rage.

As we begin to emerge from the shadows, we feel different, we are not who we were; we might look the same, but we are resonating differently now in the world. The threads of identity of who we were are looser now and we are getting used to the new threads in our tapestry.

This process was visible in a shamanic journey I received during my menopausal initiation.

> I am playing hide and seek with trolls. I am at the top of the mountain, and I see a raven and her nest. I ask if I can take a chick, she says yes, for a bit. I put it in my pocket and return to my hut.

71

> The bird grows big and I look into its eye and fall into a deep dark
> void. I then see trolls or similar rebuilding from broken crockery
> I've swept up. They build new structures that are unusual, unfamil-
> iar and out of the ordinary.

Here, we can see that I am supported by mythological beings in the form of trolls. The raven is associated with death and the underworld, yet I am at the top of the mountain, I have climbed up to the summit. There is something new forming represented by the chick. There are new structures that at this time are unfamiliar to me as they are still fragments and not fully integrated.

As we move through processing old wounds and trauma, a gentler and subtler energy becomes tangible. This can reveal itself in the form of visions, perhaps in dreams, or dream-like states or meditation. In the place where the mind rests, our inner being can express herself more clearly and we are able to hear and listen more easily. As we lie in the dark, on the riverbank, by the sea or by the oak in the woodland, we may receive *cosmic downloads*—information that is given which brings us to a simple yet profound knowing. We can begin to feel a sense of expansion where previously we may have felt contracted. This is lik-ened to the season of Spring. If you recall the few days following your moon bleed you may have felt the energy of the maiden. New ideas, a new energy but still feeling a little fragile and vulnerable. It is like the emerging seed and new sapling.

As we move through menopause, we can receive insight, informa-tion, and guidance. This can be regarding the human experience and general understanding but also more specific information about our lives and next steps. This information can most easily come to us when we are still, and the mind becomes less busy with thought. The practice of meditation can be used to quieten the mind. Mornings before we have got into our daily activities can be a good time. Often meditation is taught and practised to calm the mind and body. It is also a practice where we can settle into a space that is beyond thought and to rest in the space that thought arises from, often described as consciousness. One of the difficulties with some meditation instruction can be the denial of spontaneous thoughts arising that can be from Source, or higher self or inner Guru. If during meditation we are fixed and rigid about not allowing thoughts, we can miss beautiful and insightful wisdom aris-ing. It is a paradox, as we need to quieten the mind to hear and yet if we get too caught up in controlling thought we can miss something that is a gift. The space when we sit quietly can be likened to the womb, a space that is creative and wishing to birth, offer and gift. So, we endeavour to hold the space lightly. The purpose essentially is to align with Source, Consciousness, our inner Guru. When we align with that vibration, we are open to allow and receive insight and wisdom.

The more time we can be open to this liminal place, the betwixt and between, the more we can receive and develop our capacity to listen and see. This is part of our initiation into the crone or wise woman phase of our life. You may feel drawn to divination methods such as tarot, rune stones, oracle cards, and I Ching. You may even feel inspired to create your own divination system. Here we are invited to connect to the *sybil, oracle, volva* or *seeress* and *prophetic* roles. Our agya chakra, the seat of our intuition is awakening. Interestingly during menopause, the hormones in the pituitary gland increase, the pituitary gland being linked to agya chakra or the third eye.

During this phase of the menopause, we begin to see the light at the end of the tunnel. It is not a linear process. We can feel this new energy and then move to yet another phase of low mood, anxiety, or physical symptoms. This has certainly been my experience; the cycle of initiation is ever changing and there is a need to keep adapting to the healing or information that arises at different times.

In shamanism and witchcraft, there is a saying that goes 'hold it close for a year and a day'. This keeps a new idea or vision close to your heart and creative cauldron, it is the gestation period and incuba-tion chamber. A new idea can then be protected from other energies. This can include well-meaning judgements, opinions, and assumptions received from others. Even if offered with good intentions, often when we share a new idea prematurely it can feel diluted or even squashed by the response we may receive. We all have had an experience of sharing an idea that we are enthusiastic about, only for it to be met with reasons why it isn't such a good idea and quickly feeling deflated. From this place it is difficult to keep the momentum up for the new idea to form fully and come to bear fruit. Similarly, we cannot rush or push these ideas into being. Sometimes we must wait, be patient until things can ripen, knowing that everything has its own time frame. Nature teaches us this. We can look at the bulbs or seeds that are planted and feel secure that they will grow and flower when the time is right and all the factors such as rain, sun, and soil are participating as needed to support this process. Yet, this notion is not always easy for us to hold onto about our own ideas, inspiration, and life journey.

We can have intuitive ideas but while waiting for them to emerge and grow we need to watch that we don't let our minds pick at them, beginning to seed doubt and reason ourselves out of something. It can be useful to distract ourselves, to know they are germinating in their own sweet time, trust that we can wait and that we will know when we need to move into action.

Our dreams can offer us access and guidance from our unconscious. Throughout our menopause journey we can see our dreams as a tool to process our changing internal landscape. Dreams present in symbolic language and can take time to understand. Intentional dreaming historically and to this present day has been used in spiritual traditions and mystery schools. *Oracular* or dream work offers us a way to traverse different dimensions and offer access to otherwise hidden aspects. I include a dream practice below.

During a time prior to my menopause, I was offering work in exchange for living at a women's retreat centre. I was eager to gain more awareness of women's mysteries and cycles. The place was situated in a beautiful forest in England, where deer and wild boar were commonplace. One day we were driving along on our way back to the retreat centre when we saw that a doe had been killed on the road. We stopped the car and the woman I was with asked 'do we want it?' I felt no hesitation—'yes!' My whole body was vibrating with anticipation, the feeling you get when you know you're meeting a soul appointment. I had a deep knowing that the deer was for me. We drove it back, her fur was soft and beautiful, her body still warm. Both myself and another wanted the deer, we decided to go to sleep and dream with intention for clarity about who the deer was for. That night I dreamed that I was given a new coat and someone said, 'it's too big for her now but she will grow into it.'

As we met the next morning in circle, we shared. After hearing my dream, the group acknowledged that the deer was for me. Over the next few days, I prepared the deer. I had been a vegetarian for most of my adult life so this was a huge undertaking, even when I passed a butcher I would turn away, not wanting to see or smell the bloodied bodies of the killed. Luckily there was a guest who did have experience of skinning and butchering animals. I was so grateful as he showed me how and he helped to prepare the deer. We kept some of the meat for a communal meal and the majority was given away to a local community.

I was then on my own, finding a way to stretch and tan the skin before softening it over the coming weeks through manipulation and drying in the sun. I made a ritual burial and blessing with some of the inner organs, expressing my gratitude at the deer's sacrifice. The process felt that it connected me deeply to the deer as a guide.

I already had a deep affinity with deer from my shamanic practitioner training with the Sacred Trust. During the training our group or clan was asked to dream for a clan name. I dreamed the name 'Clan of the Running Deer' and so we were named. The deer is alert, curious, adaptable, a symbol of heart chakra.

It is only recently that I have understood that this message was for now—the new coat is about my second initiation, my moving into wise woman phase. I needed to change so I was a good fit to the qualities and gifts of the deer. This is a theme about purpose and service explored further in Chapter 8, 'Weaving the Golden Thread'.

One of the things I have learnt is to pay real attention to my own energy and follow it. This includes when I do things and when I wait. If I have an action or task to do during my day, I wait until I feel my inner energy resonates with that task. In this way I feel more satisfied, aligned, authentic, and efficient. Sometimes this isn't possible if you have responsibilities or a specific time frame, but it is surprising how things naturally get done and happen once you begin practising this.

During the menopause journey, you may feel drawn to old traditions and crafts such as weaving, knitting, and spinning. These are some of the tools of our ancestors. They have a twofold function, firstly to make useful things and secondly as an energetic creative channel or tool. When we do such activities, they naturally lend themselves to magic or energetic work. Like meditation they support us in connecting with the space beyond the egoic mind. We can, for example, spin with an intention to spin ourselves into a new beginning, or weave together new relationships or healing for ourselves or others. Old stories tell of spinning rough material usually flax into gold.[8] The spindle or distaff transforms raw fleece into thread. Interestingly the name for unmarried woman, often associated with a witch or wise woman is 'spinster'. The term *distaff* is used for anything pertaining to women and conveys woman's innate alchemical nature.

---

[8] Tom Tit Tot is the English variant of the Rumpelstiltskin fairy tale collected by Joseph Jacobs in his English Fairy Tales, published in 1890. The girl must spin flax for an entire month. (Cited by www.pookpress.co.uk accessed 15/06/22)

This phase of initiation is known as the return and corresponds to the *whiteness* of the albedo alchemical stage before moving into *rubedo*, there is a new beginning being birthed. It is like the stitching of new threads over what was a well-worn item of clothing. It becomes something new, even though it is stitched onto the foundations of the fabric underneath. It may look radically different or just have a few amendments. A new garment is created incorporating and interweaving the past, what has been outgrown, the present and has space for growth into the future.

Our physical symptoms may have abated, and we have moved into a greater acceptance of what is. We may still feel shaky, like a foal on new legs, but we are a bit more assured and rooted in ourselves once again. We may feel a little lighter and interactions with ourselves and others may seem more easeful. When we feel depleted or challenged, we are more able to traverse the landscape, we begin to feel more equipped to meet our needs.

Contemplation questions

In which ways does it help you to receive information from source? For example, through dreaming, meditation, imaging, or journaling.

Recall and reflect on how you felt during your inner spring phase of your menstrual cycle and how this correlates to your experience now.

Reflect on what occurs in nature during the season of spring.

What are the new hopes, ideas, and dreams that you are emerging with?

How are you going to protect these and encourage their growth?

What are the tools and skills that you are emerging with?

Do you feel a sense of expansion? If so, journal or image about that feeling. Refer to this when you are feeling more contracted and let it help you raise your vibration.

Practices to support your new threads

Dream intention

Before going to sleep, have clarity about what you would like to set as your intention for your dream work. Dreaming has been used in many spiritual traditions to receive information and guidance. Have your journal and pen ready by your bed.

Repeat to yourself several times your intentions, either until you feel it rooted into your consciousness or until you fall asleep. For example, 'my intention is to dream for a vision that will support me at this time' or 'my intention is to dream for information regarding my current situation'.

You may wake during the night spontaneously or in the morning. When you wake, before you do anything else, write down all that you can recall of your dream.

Reflect on the guidance you have received from a wise woman perspective from heart and womb space, rather than the rational mind. The more you work consciously with your dreams the more available your dream world will be.

When working consciously with dreamwork you may find using the herb Mugwort, as an astringent tea or in herbal smoking mix, may also assist with creativity and clarity.

Medicine walk

Set time aside for a medicine walk.

Choose a time in nature and set an intention, question, or theme. It may be for healing or guidance.

Decide on a threshold point, such as a doorway into the garden or a gate.

Know that as you step through that threshold point you will begin your medicine walk and everything that you experience is part of your answer, that nature is the visible face of spirit. Any animals, plants, or people you see or feel a connection with are part of your answer.

During your medicine walk do not try and control the experience, allow it to unfold naturally.

When ready to return, walk back through your chosen threshold point, where you began.

Journal every detail of your medicine walk that you can recall. Reflect upon it and weave together the significant pieces. There may be aspects that made no sense to you or that you cannot see the relevance of, or regard as unimportant. Write them anyway and know that they may become clearer in the future. You may feel prompted to revisit your medicine walk journaling in the coming weeks or months.

Agya awakening

The agya chakra is the energy centre connected to clairvoyance, intuition, and innate wisdom. It is located in the centre of the head, but we can use the eyebrow centre as a focal or trigger point. During your menopause, you may be aware of this awakening naturally. There may be times where you experience sensations including pulsing at the eyebrow centre.

In this practice, we focus on this energy centre to help support this natural opening and expansion of agya chakra. We can synchronise awareness at agya with silently repeating the bija mantra for Goddess Saraswati. Saraswati supports us in developing our clarity, discernment, intuition, and innate wisdom. The mantra holds the vibration of the Goddess and Her qualities.

Sit in a comfortable position or lying down.

Focus your awareness on the eyebrow centre.

Begin to become aware of your natural breath and imagine, sense or visualise breathing in and out of the space between your eyebrows in towards the centre of your head. Inhale in through the eyebrow centre to the centre of the head, and exhale out.

You may visualise a colour. The colour white or indigo is often associated with agya but work with whatever colour naturally arises for you.

Begin to repeat the bija mantra: *AIM (AI-EEM)*

Synchronise breath with mantra and awareness of agya.

Continue this practice for several minutes, resting when it feels timely to do so. When you release the practice become aware of the effects of your practice.

Externalise your awareness.

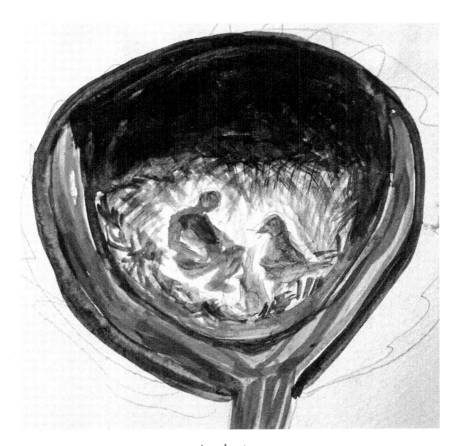

Incubation

CHAPTER 7

The Priestess is in the Temple

In our menopause rite of passage, we deepen our knowing and connection to the Priestess with the source of life. Generally, we perceive the Priestess archetype more easily than that of the witch or crone, as she has received fewer negative projections and distortions. It can be helpful to explore how these different archetypes appear for you in your personal journey and what resistances, assumptions, and conditioning you have about each.

The Priestess archetype embodies the shadowy world of the unseen world and the unconscious. In many ways, she encapsulates the menopausal state. In the Greek myth, the Queen of the Underworld is Persephone and she rules over the mysteries of the land of the dead. She is the daughter of Demeter, the Goddess of fruitfulness, earth and ripe grain. Persephone leaves behind her innocence and youth to become the guardian of the secrets of the underworld. She is linked to the inner world, the landscape that the menopause invites us to explore and know intimately. The world around us, that of daylight, youthful enthusiasm and the masculine cannot understand the world we are traversing. This archetype embodies knowledge of the invisible and primitive, we recognise ourselves as Persephone through our experiences, insights, dreams, visions and intuition. In Chapter 3, 'The Underworld', we explored the challenges of this time and the call to drop deeply into Her arms, to surrender to the pain of exquisite undoing.

In the Mythic Tarot (1995) the High Priestess is explained:

> "… having learnt something of *her* physical nature and needs and *her* place in the world … *she* now enters the night-world and comes, often with confusion and bewilderment, to that silent figure who embodies Mother on another deeper and subtler level- the womb of the unconscious in which the secret of *her* real purpose and the pattern of *her* destiny are contained."
>
> (Sharman-Burke, Greene L, 1995)

When in an intimate relationship with another, we can sometimes test the solidity and capacity of the masculine or Shiva energy to stand, hold, and contain us and our partner can feel overwhelmed or even frightened, attacked, and criticised and wants to back off. This can be experienced as weakness and rejection, eventually leading to disappointment and mistrust. Generally, women need to know that Shiva is there and can be relied upon. This lack of presence to our need can lead to further fury and alienation (Deida, 2017). Increased awareness of this dynamic can really help navigate this for both for you and your partner.

Talking and exploring the patterns that tend to happen whilst not being in that situation can really help when you are in a particular dynamic. It's a bit like having a strategy or approach in place before an avalanche or tornado—you are not caught so unawares and it's easier to flow with nature's expression. To love and appreciate the wildness without getting taken out by it, and of course, knowing it will pass. Menopause calls for the Priestess to step up and take responsibility for her communication and action, she knows that she has an impact on the world around her. She has awareness of being a conductor, director, and a deliberate creator.

As we journey through the menopause, we drop downwards but also fill out. We fill out energetically into ourselves, becoming more authentically who we are despite our conditioning. We integrate what we have gleaned from our underworld journey with our skills from the ordinary, material world.

We also fill out physically. During the menopause phase we have to process and accept the changes to our body. Wrinkles, grey hair, sagging flesh, shape change, and weight gain. For some women this can be easeful, welcoming the grey and the softer folds of flesh. Like many women, I felt that part of me has always known I would be happier as I got older, so the signs of ageing in some ways were welcomed. Body pains were less easily accepted and changes to sexual libido were also troubling. Our scent can also change; I have missed the sweet, honeyed smell of ovulation. Where once the clingy dress was certain to turn heads and open doors, we often are less confident postmenopause, and the world does not usually recognise our beauty and power.

The Priestess knows that her yoni and womb space are sacred. The Lyceum knows the universe as, *'the yoni-verse, creation itself is sweet songs of the yoni.'* (Buxton, 2004)

It feels good to keep the body juicy, the fluids vital and moving. Some women find that the use of a jade egg is a good practice. The jade egg can help maintain tone to the pelvic floor and bladder but also maintain the flow of energy in the reproductive organs. This can help prevent weakness in the bladder and avoid prolapse. The use of a jade egg can be healing and allow stuck energy or trauma to be released. Minke de Vos in *Tao Tantric Arts for Women* describes jade egg practices in detail. (Minke de Vos, 2016)

At different stages in our lives, our yoni holds on a cellular level different experiences. This can include traumatic experiences where we were not loving and caring to our bodies and yoni. There may have been times where we may have been violated, said yes when we meant no, given birth, cervical smears, hysterectomy, miscarriage, abortion, and wonderful sexual unions too.

If you are not in a relationship these themes and practices can be adapted and seen in the context that you are getting ready for a new, fulfilling relationship, if you want one. It can take more discipline to put the time aside for self-love. Often if we are not in a relationship, we have less touch and this is important to allow us to soften our bodies, feel held and supported, and sooth our nervous system.

For many women the change in physical body and the change in sexual energy can be devastating. Many women feel that if they are in a relationship, they need to be able to continue to have sex as they did so previously. If this does not feel comfortable physically or emotionally, it can lead to fear and anxieties that their partner may leave them.

During perimenopause I noticed how often my sexual energy and vibration matched that of younger men, and I could feel their confusion about what they were feeling and the thought process about me being too old for them. The irony is that for many of us we have dressed down in our lives so as not to receive unwanted sexual attention and then at midlife we miss receiving sexual attention.

With the change in hormone levels, sexual desire can reduce and you may experience vaginal dryness. You may have been content with your sexual relationship, partnership, marriage, and self-pleasuring but then like many things this may begin to not feel so good. It may even feel invasive or uncomfortable. Sadly, many women decide or assume that that's the end of sexual intimacy and passion for them. This can then lead to a decline in mood based on feeling undesired, a lack of physical contact and losing something that you may have previously found enlivening and enjoyable.

However, like many other life areas the menopause can be a time to pause, recalibrate, and reconsider, what is of value to you? What do you enjoy and want? You may feel a shift within your sexual role, a wish to explore different roles. You may wish to find new and innovative ways to touch and be touched. This exploration can lead to new, unexplored territory that can surprise and delight you and your partner if you have one.

When we allow the conditioned responses to fall away and approach our love-making with renewed curiosity, play, presence, and openness something opens up. Bringing change into love-making can feel risky, particularly if you are in a long-term relationship … Is it worth stirring the pot? Responses such as making sounds to encourage, please, affirm our partner may not be authentic, habitual patterns of foreplay may feel somewhat tired and predictable, the thrust may have lost some of its magic, and chasing the end goal of orgasm may seem less satisfying. When we let go of sexual strategy and practice, present awareness through the senses, our intimacy can deepen.

One of the beautiful ways to begin to create a new paradigm of love-making is by taking time to make the space beautiful and setting a time when you will come together in sacred union. As with all alchemy, a strong and safe container is necessary and taking time to put this in place through basic relationship housekeeping and creating a beautiful, uninterrupted space is important. This also clearly separates it from the mundane and the responsibilities of the day. It honours the union and allows you both to prepare with anticipation and be clear about what you are bringing to the shared time. You may wish to let this meeting be a ritual or a spontaneous unfurling. Spending time sitting facing one another and meeting each other's gaze for a few moments helps attune to one another.

At times it may be helpful to have a few minutes to take turns to share anything that needs to be said, so it can be cleared and set aside, allowing you to be fully present. If it feels right to you, you may honour each other as expressions of Shiva and Shakti, speaking this aloud. These simple practices can have a profound effect on the following interactions. The inner self or higher self is awake and present and can allow a beautifully refined union to emerge. The space created is that of co-creation, the coming together of both your energies to create a third energy.

In *Making Love, Sexual Love the Divine Way,* Barry Long (1998) is frank as he describes the dissonance between women and men and the unhealthy patterns of behaviour that we have learnt that prevent us from feeling deeply fulfilled and as love:

> "For to be in love and to keep love fresh and new requires tremendous awareness, tremendous presence. Be in love in this way and your love will not end, for love has no end. Fall in love and your love will end." (Long, 1989, p37)

In this inspiring book, he reminds us of our capacity for divine love and that we can start with love-making. When we endeavour to love fully and raise our consciousness through love we can give guidance and be an inspired example. The path of sacred intimacy requires deep honesty and courage and is an ongoing practice of showing up and being present.

> "For man and woman at the beginning of time were gods, and they sustained the awareness and presence of their godhead, their timelessness, by making divine physical love."

There are many ways to connect and explore together. A lovely practice is to rub oil into each other and then move together, without focusing on the erogenous areas. Touch different parts of the body, back-to-back, front, sideways, making it playful and curious, allowing the energy to rise naturally and easefully. This type of practice may lead to further intimacy and sexual sharing, or it may be enough connection in itself. It is helpful to keep checking in with one another to see where you both are with the sharing. It is no point continuing with such a practice if only one of you is engaged.

If you have been with a partner for a long time these practices can bring welcome refreshment to the bedroom. Often, we get stuck in patterns of touching and as we change, these patterns can become unwelcome and disharmonising, often having the opposite effect to what was intended!

Another practice that is beautiful is to place a mantra into your body or your partner's body. This is an adaptation of an ancient tantric practice called *nyasa,* where a mantra is placed within different parts of the body. If you are familiar with the chakras then this can be a lovely place to start. You might ask your partner to place the Shakti mantra *HRIM* at each chakra or energy wheel. Or you may like to place the mantra *AUM* at specific points on your partner's body. If you feel unfamiliar with mantra then any word that resonates with love, respect, devotion can be used. For example, touching your partner's forehead and saying aloud *'I place love here, because that is who you are'.*

In our sexual lives, many of us have grown de-sensitised to touch. Sometimes a subtle touch is barely noticed, and we crave bolder, firmer touch. Of course, there is nothing wrong with this but if it comes from a place of being cut off, trauma, or habit, it can be sweet to explore different types of touch. This may include stroking yourself or your partner with a feather or a fingertip, you can experiment with pressure and speed. These practices support us in moving away from erotic zone focus. Often, we can get into the habit of taking shortcuts, 'she likes me to touch her breast for a bit, then clitoris, then I can penetrate' or 'if I make pleasurable sounds and touch his cock he will be happy', can be common habitual scripts. Maintaining eye contact during lovemaking can be challenging as we are fully seen and in doing so are vulnerable. We stay in the present moment rather than drifting into fantasy. We see our partner and we are seen.

For heterosexual couples, when the lingam is inside the yoni, it is aligned with specific meridian points that correspond to our internal organs (Minke de Vos, 2016). When we explore the lingam being still inside the yoni it can bring deep healing, as well as cascades of pleasure and delight. When allowed to relax, the sexual organs begin to talk to one another. For this communication to be able to happen we need to move beyond our sexual conditioning of focusing on the thrust and orgasm. This can be very challenging for both partners, but the practice can be fun and enjoyable. If we can get out of the way we have the potential to enter a shared space of spontaneous awareness where deep healing and pleasure can take place on every level.

Just as it is not helpful to push and grasp at ideas, projects, or things you want in your life, similarly during love-making if we can surrender and let go of preconceived ideas about foreplay and orgasm, we can open to divine love-making. Here we allow a greater presence to move through us and guide us.

> "It's the dissolution or death of self that gives rise to true passion."
> (Long, 1998, p27)

In most, if not all, religious and spiritual traditions, there is an energetic or esoteric branch and in these, they agree that sexual energy has much potential not only as way to connect deeply to the divine and each other but also to transform. By moving our focus away from lust, passion, and orgasmic outcome, we transmute the energy into that which can transform. Don't get me wrong I am all for expressions of primal lust and passion when desired, but this is a life phase which naturally lends itself to exploring sacred sexuality. The Priestess knows that sacred sexuality is a doorway into embracing the Divine. As our libido changes this is one of the gifts of the initiation.

Historically, the Priestess would also have had a role in educating young women and men into the art of love-making. In many cultures sacred prostitution was revered and honoured, there was an acknowledgement of the beauty and artistry in intimacy and the potential for touching and merging with the divine through our sensual bodies. We have moved so far away from this knowing, but at this time of the re-emergence of the sacred feminine there is a gentle remembering. As wise women we are well placed to recall and retrieve these ancient teachings. Mary Magdalene has been depicted as a common whore by the patriarchy whom Jesus saved. Yet, increasingly she is being remembered as an accomplished initiate of women's mystery schools and as a mistress of sacred intimacy and Priestess. In *The Magdalene Manuscripts*, Tom Kenyan and Judi Sion [2002] describe how she was an initiate in the traditions of Isis and Horus and that it was through her spiritual advancement and accomplishment that Yeshua or Jesus was supported to accomplish his soul's purpose.

"The sexual magic of Isis has to do with the innate ability of the feminine being to utilise the magnetic energies to open deeper levels of consciousness through the act of surrendering to the sexual energies and pathways that are opened." (Kenyan, Sion, 2002)

You and your partner enter the temple of intimacy and you step into the role of Priestess. In your power, sensual and aware of the energy flowing within yourself and between you and your partner, tune in, adjust, and adapt to the situation before you. What is needed in your co-creation? What do you and your partner need and desire? Part of this phase is to allow time to create the space but also feel into where you both are. You and your partner may wish to take plenty of time to let the energy and juices flow before any penetration or allow the lingam and yoni to guide the union, where an erect lingam is not necessary. Love-making becomes an art form, a co-creation, and dance of the sacred feminine and sacred masculine.

"The purpose of the lovemaking is served when the divine energies have been gathered". (Long, 1998, p53)

The energies are gathered, not to create new physical life as when we are in our maternal phase of life, but rather to bring heightened capacity to hold energy and love. We have a deep yearning to let go and surrender into love. This being our desire to return from separation with the Divine to union. During intimacy, as with other practices, such as meditation and dance, we can experience this union. Often fear can hold us back from truly softening and letting go. Deida describes this beautifully,

"Nothing outside of us has the power to limit our capacity to give and receive love ... It is a choice, a practice ... unbind the knots we have tightened around our heart so we can live free as love". (Deida, 2004)

During this life phase and alchemical stage of the philosopher's stone, the inner desire to integrate and balance your feminine and masculine qualities can become more pronounced. The left brain that deals with focus, action, assertiveness, striving, and linear thought is associated with masculine essence and the right brain that of intuition, care, empathy, love, and beauty associated with feminine essence. You may explore holding the masculine, allowing your partner to lean into you, allowing their gentle and more vulnerable and receptive aspects. We want to encourage and develop a positive and strong relationship between the right and left sides of our brain.

Alchemically, the image of a sexual couple is used to illustrate the third stage, where opposites are integrated in a new way. During my menopause initiation, I found myself drawn to practices and movements that helped to balance these two parts of the brain. Using opposite or diagonal movements help this and they also help maintain balance of body and mind. Using your less dominant hand to do things like brushing your teeth or eating your meal and exploring being ambidextrous can be interesting. I also found my art making, visions, and dreams began exploring the union between male and female.

This integration not only helps us be in balance physically, emotionally, and energetically, it can also have a practical function. Often women have been trained and consented to being dependent on the masculine. Many women I know have no understanding of their finances, car, boiler, or mortgage in their shared lives as their role has been to focus on the homemaking and the children's needs. This stereotypical polarity in roles can work beautifully for some heterosexual couples but for others there can be an increased feeling of dependency and not utilising their own intellect and feeling disempowered. This of course also can happen the other way, the man feeling equally closed off from his feminine essence making it the harder for him to share deeply about his emotional needs and concerns. This dynamic also can be at play in same sex relationships where individuals are identifying strongly with either masculine or feminine qualities. As we have increased awareness of our social conditioning and take more responsibility for our healing, integrating both feminine and masculine aspects, we are more able to traverse and flow with the changes and transitions in life.

The sacred glyph or symbol known as *lemniscate*, the infinity symbol depicted as the figure of eight, is an important symbol for this time in our process. Not only as we traverse our own menopause but also in our evolution at this time. This is the *lemniscus infinitorum*, the dance of infinite flight (Buxton, 2004). This is the waggle dance that bees use to communicate with each other about colony or hive business. The symbol is comprised of two orbs and a knot at the centre where they meet. This symbol holds the polarities and duality of life. It is central in the Lyceum, which is a gynocentric shamanic tradition. In this tradition, the honeybee is a sacred ally. One of the ways that the bees communicate is through the use of this symbol. The lemniscate, when used in our practice, helps us integrate and assimilate the polarities that we hold. This can include feminine and masculine essence. It can also be worked with the sun and moon, light and dark, and so on. There are many ways to practice with this symbol, it can open us up to multi-dimensional realms. Experiment with moving this around your body (see practices below). As we integrate polarities in a new, deep level we are opening up to a new state, a new dawn.

We have been taught that we need to have a fulfilling relationship to be happy. We have learnt that this relationship is with someone else. We have been taught that we should bend and facilitate this, often at all costs, if we wish to be loved and accepted. As we mature and through our menopause journey, we become more rooted in the knowing that the most important relationship is with ourselves. All of ourselves, the higher, inner being and the egoic manifest aspects of our being. As we build a good relationship with ourselves, we are able to stand more fully in our power with kindness and compassion to ourselves and others.

As we move towards the final phases of menopause, we step into our sovereignty, having gained increased clarity about our place in the world. We are no longer dependent or submissive to conditioned roles and assumptions, no longer adapting our lives to please others and feel worthy. We have met out intrinsic worthiness and unique goodness. We can step into our power. We have evaluated what drains our energy and what enhances it and consciously make choices to move towards alignment and a positive, enhancing energy and vibration. We are aware of our wounds but not paralysed or re-traumatised by them. We are aware of our edges and boundaries and have the confidence to maintain them. We can stand at the centre of who we are and have a strong sense of self and connection with the natural world around us.

The Priestess knows that the sacred is hidden in the mundane. For centuries women have concealed their magic and power. Partly due to the systematic and consistent subjugation of women and the societal roles that governed them. As women had the role of homemakers and had little independence, they connected to the Divine by weaving it into their daily lives. This included approaching tasks, however small, boring, mundane, unpleasant, from a spiritual perspective. When we stay connected to our inner being, our heart space, our knowing that everything is an expression of the Divine we are more able to keep mind focused and spacious. This then lends itself to using any tasks as a practice. This can be used with any functional task and was by our ancestors, such as sweeping, cooking or cleaning. For example, when cleaning windows you can have the intention that you are removing that which clouds your perception about ageing, when washing up you can wash away your grief or shame. The profound is often in the simple and mundane.

The Melissae, the Sisterhood of the Hive and the Priestesses within the Greek temples are linked with the Oracle at Delphi. Delphi was a centre for pilgrimage in ancient classical his-her-story. People came to the oracle at the temple to receive Divine guidance. The appearance of a swarm of bees heralded the oracle's arrival. The Priestesses of Eleusis were also known as Melissae and their temple known as the beehive. One of the likely functions of the Priestess was to transmute ordinary bodily secretions into healing *nektars* or elixirs. Likewise, in the Shakti and tantric traditions the Priestess or yogini knows that her body is the temple and alchemical vessel. Menopause invites us to embody and integrate our spirituality thoroughly and unashamedly.

> "Returning the scenes, desires, passions and sexuality to the spiritual being is the most profound and the most audacious inner adventure ever imagined." (Odier, 1999)

During the menopause, we are harmonising our mooladhara chakra, the energy centre of home, roots, security. This is what is shaken during perimenopause. As our sexual energy shifts, we are also working with swadithana, the pelvic energy centre. This is represented by half a reptile and half dolphin, another example of the hybrid, the shapeshifter. This is our sexual centre, our sensory desire, our unconscious, deep emotions, linked to element of water. As we change in these domains of home, security, sexuality, sensuality, and creativity, we bring our energy to manipur chakra and how we are in the world. It is our new or modified version of our old self and when our initiation is completing, we prepare to venture back out into the world.

This can be a time where you can tune into the lineage of Priestesses to guide you. Many women feel called to connect with Mary Magdalene at this time. We keep our intention to keep an open and tender heart despite the experiences we may have had. This is the path of the spiritual warrior, the Priestess in her glory—to have the courage to keep on loving.

Contemplation questions

What is your relationship to the Priestess archetype?

How do you feel about your body changing?

How has your sexual energy changed during your life? Reflect back through your teens, twenties, thirties, and forties until now.

How do you wish to be touched at this time, if at all?

How do you feel about touching yourself?

How is your relationship with yourself? How could this feel even better?

If you are in a sexual relationship, are you satisfied? If not, what would you like to change?

Do you identify mainly with feminine or masculine essence? How could you integrate the other more within yourself?

In which ways do you give and receive—is one more dominant in your life?

How is your heart? How can you keep softening and loving?

Practices to support the Priestess

Infinity breath

Practice with a partner or friend.

Join hands, allowing a cross where your wrists meet. This being the central knot. Your eyes can gently close.

Gently imagine, sense the energy moving around the infinity symbol, each person at the centre of an orb. Allow the body to sway gently if this occurs naturally, allow yourself to tune in and follow the energy. This may be slow or become faster, allow the experience to come from the inside out rather than from the outside in.

When it feels right, pause at the centre, then move in the other direction, then pause again. Release the practice and sit with the effects of the practice. Take your time to externalise your awareness.

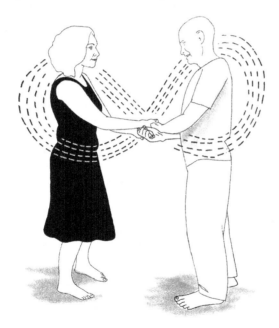

Infinity with couple

Sacred in the mundane

Choose a mundane task that you do every day, preferably one that you don't particularly like or is so habitual you don't even think about it. For example, washing up, cleaning your teeth, getting dressed, hoovering, driving to work. Set an intention that for seven days you will do this task with full awareness and as a sacred act. You may wish to cultivate gratitude or devotion as you complete your task. Observe how your relationship and feeling about this task changes.

Alternate nostril breathing

Alternate nostril breathing or *nadi shodhana* (also known as psychic network purification) is a pranayama practice. Pranayama is ideally learnt in person with a teacher; it is important never to strain and to stop the practice if you feel any adverse side effects. This practice is wonderful during menopause as it brings balance to both the left and right sides of the brain. This includes the energy channels within the body known as *nadis,* particularly ida and pingula that correspond with the masculine/feminine, sun/moon energies. It helps reduce anxiety, balances the nervous system, and improves concentration (Satyananda, 1969).

Sit in a comfortable seated posture with the spine upright. Relax the body and bring your awareness to your natural breath.

You will be using a hand position or *mudra* for this practice. Raise your right arm and have your thumb by the right nostril and your ring finger by your left nostril, *nasagra mudra.* The other fingers can relax or lightly place the index and middle fingers to rest on your eyebrow centre.

Close the right nostril with the thumb and inhale through the left nostril. Close the left nostril and breath out through the right nostril. Count the number it is comfortable to inhale and exhale without strain. Continue in this way working towards the ratio of 1:1, an equal inhalation and exhalation. For example, a count of four as you inhale and a count of four as you exhale. With practice, you will find that your breath will become longer.

You may then practice with the ratio of 1:2, the inhalation being half the count of the exhalation. Maintain a relaxed attitude and allow no strain.

After 5–10 rounds, sit and become aware of the benefit of your practice. Externalise your awareness.

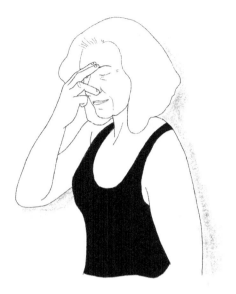

Alternate nostril breathing

Massage (solo)

Take time to prepare your space. Make sure the space is warm so your body can relax, light a candle and incense if that pleases you.

Use some olive oil, sesame oil, or other oil of your choosing. Add some essential oil if you wish—a nice option is rose, you might also make your own blend. Warm the oil by standing it in a bowl of hot water for a few moments.

Gently massage the oil into your skin, feel the pleasure of the contact and the warmth of the oil. Take your time and luxuriate, connecting to yourself as an embodiment of the Goddess. Be aware of any resistance to this and contemplate where it arises from.

Sensory ceremony (couple)

This is a beautiful practice, adapted from *The Art of Sexual Ecstasy* by Margo Anand (1991). It can really increase the heartfelt connection between you as a couple. If you are in partnership with a man, to offer this devotion to him can be very healing for the masculine wounds. In my experience, on some level men know that the wounded feminine resents them and is angry and that they have failed to show up as fully as we need them at times. Arguably, they also have felt threatened and intimidated by the power of woman and her capacity to love deeply and create life. So, when we offer such unconditional, love, acceptance, and devotion to him it can be a profound experience. The phrase *penis envy* is now used in mainstream culture and yet *womb envy* is not. This concept, that of envying and therefore fearing and wishing to destroy the infinite intelligence, power and life-giving creative capacity of woman, can be regarded as being at the root of patriarchy and the persistent and systematic subjugation of women. As women we are invited to offer compassion and understanding towards these wounds. This practice and others like it can provide a safe space for this healing to occur.

Make sure that you won't be disturbed, and you have no time limit of the session together. Decide who will be receiving and who giving. For this description I will assume the woman is holding the temple space for a male partner. Take time to prepare the space making it a beautiful temple. Use your imagination and your inner Priestess to guide you to create a beautiful sacred space that is worthy of the Divine. You may wish to play music that enhances the mood, use incense, rose petals, and candles.

Choose a selection of objects to offer the senses, smells, tastes, touch, and sounds. This may include small bells, fresh rosemary, honey, chocolate, a feather. Place them on a tray.

Ask your partner to come at the agreed time and know that verbal communication will drop away during the ceremony. Before they enter the space make eye contact letting him know that they can trust you and that this is a space for him to let go and receive fully, you can then use a scarf to blindfold him. We rest the sense of sight to allow an increased use and appreciation of our other senses. Lead him gently into the space and help him find a seat on a chair or rugs and cushions.

Without rushing, one by one introduce him to a sensory experience that you have prepared. You may run a feather along his leg, ask him to gently open his mouth to receive a small piece of chocolate, smell the scent of the essential oils. Take your time. Allow him to shift from left brain thinking to right brain receiving. It may help to massage his shoulders, feet or stroke his face if he is finding it hard to relax and trust.

When you have finished offering him the sensory experience you can hold him in your arms, allow his body to relax and be supported by you. Make sure you feel supported yourself with cushions, chair or wall. If it feels right in the moment, you may hum to him.

During the practice, be attentive to his being yet also to your own energy. Notice if you lose yourself whilst you are in service. Practice maintaining your own grounded presence and being in your own energy field at the same time as offering your service and devotion.

Close the session with Grace and gratitude. Take your time to leave the temple atmosphere. On another day exchange roles or create a similar ceremony.

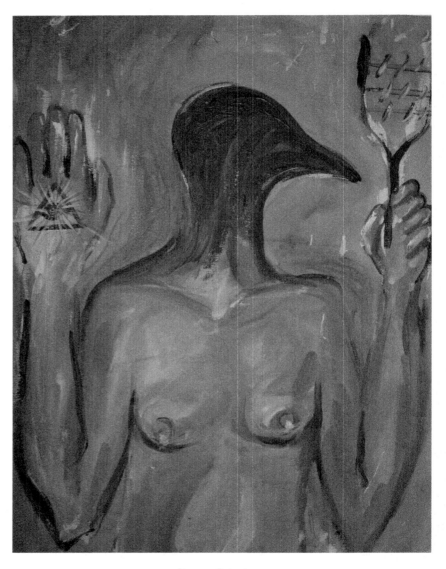

Raven Priestess

CHAPTER 8

Weaving the Golden Thread

It is a strange experience moving towards your last bleed; I felt that each and every bleed was precious, I wanted to have more blood as it dwindled. I was even more particular at using it; on the garden, ingesting, in ritual, ceremony and painting with it are all ways that we can appreciate and use it. Science is beginning to confirm (Rodrigues, 2016) what the wise woman knows and is doing more research into the healing potential of menstrual or moon blood. It contains a particular form of stem cells, these are the cells that form and sustain new life, they come from the womb of creation and birth.

As discussed in Chapter 1, 'Red River Runs Dry', this loss can be huge for many women. It can particularly bring up any unresolved issues about not having born children, or fear and anxiety about who you will be if you are not a mother or potential mother. It can be unsettling if you are a woman who has followed your moon's rhythm—the seasons of your body—with conscious awareness. With this guiding rhythm gone, it's as if the rudder on your boat is broken and you're out at sea. Yet, the moon continues with Her waxing and waning, and we can shift our attention to that rhythm and cycle. As our red river runs dry, we enter the alchemical stage of *rebedo*, the red gold stage. As the indigenous oral teaching states, 'we hold our wise blood on the inside', our crucible now contains the essence within rather than releasing it outwards.

I have noticed that around the dark moon some of my symptoms intensify, the body aches more, social communication is more of an effort. This is much like my autumn and winter when I was bleeding. So, we begin to notice new patterns or old patterns in a new way.

Without the moon bleed cycle to navigate, we can feel into and listen even more acutely to our own energy patterns. Is this the time to visit family or friends? Is this the time to create or rest? We can also use the moon's cycle to make resolutions or to make offerings or perform a ritual. On a new moon you may set a new intention for yourself, harnessing this new energy for new ideas and projects. Or you may wish to work with the full moon energy, where things have waxed and ripened, when they are at their fullest. This is a good time to make a pledge and an offering. This could be personal prayer or for the collective and greater good. In doing so, we work with and harness the cosmic energies.

When we weave our golden thread, we weave our new visions, insights, and dreams into our new world or reality. This is where the subtle and solid qualities of our new state of being are woven and integrated. This is the *rubedo* and philosopher's stone, the final alchemical stage—where lead is transmuted to gold.

In Greek mythology, the Lyceum tradition and other spiritual traditions, the three fates, Norns, Wyrd Sisters, or Moirai are teachers and hold rich symbology. They signify the three Goddesses and stages of a woman's life. Moirai means 'a phase', and the moon has three phases and three aspects: the new moon, corresponds to the maiden, Goddess of spring. The full moon, relates to the mother, Goddess of the summer and the second phase of life. The dark moon, corresponds to the crone or wise woman, the Goddess of autumn and winter, the final phase of life. The three fates have different tasks that relate to our human destiny, the first being Clotho the spinner, spinning her thread on a golden spindle. The second Lachesis who measures the length of the thread of a life and Atropos the cutter of that thread, 'she who cannot be avoided' (Greene, 1995). These Sisters remind us that spinning and weaving has long been associated with women's mysteries in all cultures.

"Behind the wheel stand the Moirai, and there is an intelligent and orderly plan behind the apparently random changes in life. These ancient figures are within us, deep in the womb of the unconscious ..." (Greene, 1995)

The wheel of the spinning wheel symbolises the cyclical wheel of life. A wheel has no beginning and no end. The three fates weave the thread of life, including the destiny, once woven it cannot be changed. They reside in the dark, in the shadows of a cave which represents the womb of Mother Earth.

For the Greeks, Athena was the goddess of spinning and weaving and in the story of the Minotaur in Crete, Ariadne gave Theseus a ball of thread which would lead him back out of the Labyrinth. In the Celtic tradition of 'The Prophecies of Merlin' Ariadne is the weaver, who directs a triple thread from her distaff, of time, space, and energy. In ancient textiles, a highly charged symbol language was used to communicate her story and myth. Spinning and weaving were imbued with magic powers and in many traditions the spider is the Great Weaver of life. This is particularly so in the tradition of Navaho blanket creation. It is considered that Spider Woman was working through the individual weaver who directed the growth of the blanket, and baby girls were prepared by a special ritual for their future as weavers (Dunbar, 2007).

As I was nearing the end of my time in the woods, I was clearing away the sweat lodge following the ceremony the night before. I fell into a liminal space and as I moved the rocks that create and hold the heat within the lodge, I experienced them as dragon's eggs. One by one I cradled them as I moved them to be stored for the following dark moon. As I carried them, I felt myself shapeshift into an elder woman, I sensed a dragon around the space, watching and breathing into me the knowing that I was becoming a *wisdom keeper*. I was carrying something of value. In the Celtic tradition, the dragon symbolises power and wisdom. The dragon, like the bee and the serpent, is often a gatekeeper to other worlds and guardian of treasures. The dragon is also linked to fire, they can scorch and burn, but this dragon breathed smoke not fire, perhaps a symbol that I had moved through the climax of my menopause initiation.

Cross-culturally eggs are a symbol of hope and new beginnings. In many spiritual traditions, the golden egg is a symbol of cosmic wholeness. In Hinduism, the golden egg, golden womb or universal womb (*Hiranyagarbha*), is the seed of all existence and is found in several ancient images and texts from Indus Valley and the Vedas (Bake, 2018). Postmenopause we incubate our cosmic or spiritual eggs within our energetic womb space. With our intention we incubate them, sustaining them with the golden thread we are learning to spin and weave into a new reality. As we move through our menopausal rite of passage we are invited to step up and even if we don't know what that means or looks like, we willingly engage with the process. Part of us can feel unworthy, ill-equipped, unready and yet we are the ones that pave the way for the women and men to follow. We take our fledgling steps forwards into crone-dom.

> "The woman who is willing to make that change must become pregnant with herself at last." (Mankowitz, 1984, p109)

What an interesting concept, to carry ourselves, to be pregnant with ourselves at last, allowing the growth and newness to develop. It feels very different to hold this in your vibration rather than to hold the thoughts and associated feelings of 'being past it'.

As we move into postmenopause, we begin to see the magic in everyday life increasingly, the synchronicities, the power of our thoughts and their vibrations mirrored into our reality. We begin to step back more, to witness and allow younger women to step up, supporting them. We are moving into a teacher role, knowing that others are following us and that we can aspire to be the role model that we perhaps didn't have. This is not always easy, we can feel the tug of competition or envy, sometimes that's the way it is. I have been aware of women in my life seeming to not be encouraging me to shine—it can take a lot of resolve to go beyond what we ourselves received. Sometimes we can and other times we may not be able to, but we gently and loosely hold that desire and intention.

We choose to spin our golden thread and make beautiful things with our thoughts, words and actions. Of course, you may have already been doing this before perimenopause but for many of us, it isn't until we have journeyed through menopause and settle into postmenopause that we begin to gain clarity and vision about our place in the world. We may begin to feel that we are leaving the priestess behind and relate more to the crone or wise woman archetype.

Some women have clarity about their purpose in the world and others reach menopause still with the question on their lips, 'what is my purpose?' Your purpose may change, or you may move through menopause and still not have that clarity. Sometimes the answer is not given in the way we expected. Rather than have clarity that your purpose is to be a helicopter pilot or herbalist it may be more about the qualities or essence that you inhabit as you continue to walk in life. To keep desiring and expanding, to keep an open heart, to breath, to follow energy rather than 'shoulds' and linear thinking. You may have insights about how you wish to serve in an expansive community-focused way rather than from an individualised perspective. Our new sense of ourselves emerges as we return and we either know or ask 'how can I be in service to others and the whole? How do I meet my soul's purpose?'

The Lyceum speaks of the Queen bee, 'she is as a goddess whose life is dedicated to selfless service within the dim light of the golden city.' In yoga, selfless service or karma yoga[9] is also central to our growth and evolution. We may find that this concept is useful as we shape our crone years.

Postmenopause, which is medically defined as one year following our last bleed, we become increasingly aware that we need to speak our truth and be authentic in how we live our lives. Even if we have done plenty of healing during our lives and specifically during our menopause journey, at times we can still feel risk and fear when speaking and living our truth. When we put ourselves out there, we are faced with old scripts, such as 'who does she think she is?', 'what of value do I have to gift?'. These fears may be born from not only our conditioning as women but can also arise from remembered experiences of when we previously were persecuted for expressing ourselves. Historically, to speak about women's mysteries would often have led to being ostracised, incarcerated, punished and even executed. This relates to how difficult it still can be for us as women to share our wisdom and authenticity. Unfortunately, we can still be met with less than encouragement from both women and men when we venture forth with our gifts. As I was writing this book, those fears arose, a primitive, illogical vibration held deep in my cells.

The centre for communication and expression is the thyroid and energetically, vishuddhi chakra. We can speculate that the reason so many women have thyroid related conditions is in relation to this historical persecution. Some women feel it so strongly, it's as if a seal has been placed on the thyroid preventing full expression of themselves. It can be helpful to work with practices that awaken and balance the chakras, particularly the throat chakra and also manipur and anahat chakras

---

[9]Karma yoga is the yogi practice of selfless service; you perform a task without any expectation of reward or acknowledgement. The action is performed without the ego's preferences being expressed.

when developing our capacity to express ourselves fully. Manipur being the energy centre related to our presence and will in the world. Anahat chakra relates to our heart centre and the qualities of compassion, love, and empathy. By bringing into harmony and strength these three chakras we are more able to communicate authentically from a place of heart into the world.

The wise woman mysteries belong to us all. The patriarchy led us to believe that only certain people had the authority to hold wisdom and spiritual or sacred space. This is not true; we are called to step up and remember our innate sacred wisdom, our capacity to heal ourselves, others, and our environment.

With this awareness comes an increased capacity to intentionally create or manifest. Whether this comes as an aspect of your menopause journey or at another time, it is a beautiful perspective (Hicks, 2004). One of the Universal Laws is the law of attraction—what we focus on we attract more of to ourselves. The universe responds to vibration, so, whether we focus on what is wanted or not wanted, it does not matter. The strength of the vibration is activating. Generally, we think similar thoughts, and this continues a repetition of events and interactions in our lives. We build up stories and then have expectations about how things will work out, and as we hold that vibration, they meet that expectation. As we intentionally create, we know that we have more mastery (or miss-stery) over our reality and what we manifest, things are not put down to happenstance. Esther Hicks (2004) teaches that when we hold a vibration of something for about seventeen seconds it is activated without resistance and gains enough momentum to change our vibration. When we connect to a vibration that is uplifting and feels good, we are tuning into that and aligning to that vibrational frequency, which will invite more of the same. We don't need to get into specifics about what we desire or need, just practice focusing on good feeling states. When you sit quietly, you can recall a state, a feeling of satisfaction, fun, and happiness. When we allow ourselves to bathe in that vibration it is becoming our predominant vibrational energy and the universe will match it. In the initiation phase of menopause, we have increased focus and clarity on the abundance we wish to create, how we wish to live the remainder of our lives and intentionally creating can support us in this. This may include abundance on a material level and an expansion of virtues or qualities for ourselves and globally. We have more discipline and skill in our thinking, or at least we can hold the intention to keep developing this capacity.

You may emerge from your menopause with changes on different levels. Your relationships and friends, your career. Some women start a whole new phase, setting up a new business or venture, you may move home, your priorities may have shifted. As we change internally our outer world follows. We are taught that our inner world is based on our outer world, we probably believed the myth that if you study hard, work hard, get married, and have children you will be rewarded with abundance and happiness. For some this has played out truthfully, but for many women and men this is a false story that is dismantled once and for all during menopause.

If we are in a space where we are unsure about our purpose, whether this follows the role of motherhood or not, it can be useful to reflect upon the other creative projects in your life. When I did this, I realised how many lovely and satisfying projects I have given birth to. This helped me hold in mind that postmenopause I would also continue to create and give birth to other projects that will satisfy myself and others. Often when we are self-orientated, women are called selfish. Yet, when we are attending to our own needs, we are then able to share in meaningful and generous ways.

Through this rite of passage our external world changes to match the internal landscape that has emerged. There can be a sense of renewal and a welcoming of the new self. When I have asked postmenopause women about their experience and where the 'gold' was for them, they describe it as a *being* rather than a *trying*, a greater ability to relax and be in the here and now. A spiritual focus and dimension opens up for them on the other side of the metamorphosis of menopause. Whilst still in the process, like the honeybee, we trust that the nectar can and will become honey. With increased awareness we weave our honeyed golden threads into cloth fit for the sovereign Queen that we are and continue to become. One side of the cloth is gold and the other infinite, velvet blackness. It is in this blackness that we see clearly and connect to Source with greater ease. Both the black and the gold make up the whole cloth, stitched and integrated together.

The greatest thread is the umbilical cord, this cord attaches us to our birth mother and gives us life. As we move through our menopause initiation, we know that we are now connected to the cosmos, to the Great

Mother via a thread or cord that is unconditional, sustaining and loving and cannot be severed.

As we navigate our passage, we enter the Queendom of the Heart. The heart is the centre of our expansion as love, reflected in many of the spiritual teachings. Banafsheh Sayyad (2022) the Sufi dancer, says that we hear a call to love and that love is a state of being not an emotion. We all have our own unique journey to make to awakening or coming 'home'. Through our journey we must continue to find the courage to keep loving and trust in the transformative power of our nature.

Contemplation questions

🖋 What shape are you weaving your golden thread into being? This may be clear or a whisper that is still forming.

🖋 How might you cherish, support, and spin this golden thread?

🖋 What do your new seeds or dragon or golden eggs need for incubation, fertilisation, and birthing?

🖋 What are the resistances, fears, and blocks that may hold you back from sharing your gifts?

🖋 Do you feel ready to celebrate and honour the journey of menopause that you have traversed? If so, how would you like this to be? If not, what do you need currently on your journey?

🖋 What have you learnt through this initiation?

🖋 What changes have you made, internally and in physical, manifest reality?

🖋 In what ways have your priorities to yourself and others changed?

🖋 How do you wish to step into being an elder, wisdom keeper, seer, grandmother, crone, and wise woman?

🖋 What new story are you weaving?

Practices to honour your golden thread

Vishuddhi awakening

Sit or lie down in a comfortable position.

Become aware of the natural breath. Imagine, sense, or visualise the breath at the throat centre. Inhaling into the throat and exhaling out.

You may imagine the breath at vishuddhi chakra as a light blue colour.

As you continue to breathe, hold the intention to release and clear any old held fears around communication and expressing your truth. With each exhalation allow any of these old energies to be released.

Continue for 5–20 minutes.

Release the practice and externalise your awareness.

Invoking Goddess Lakshmi

Sit in a comfortable position.

Allow the spine to lift and a sense of grounding down toward the earth through your sitting bones.

Become aware of the air and space around the body and above the head.

Become aware of your natural breath, the body inhaling and the body exhaling.

Bring to mind the image of Goddess Lakshmi, wearing white. She has four arms and is holding a vena (guitar type instrument). Golden coins fall from her palm, and she is holding a gold cup of abundance in one hand and a lotus flower in the other. She is with a white swan. As you visualise her begin to feel her qualities of abundance, contentment, love, and joy.

Hold in mind the qualities that you would like to develop at this time, perhaps the intention to hold abundance and love in your heart.

Repeat the mantra *OM SHRIM LAKSHMYAI NAMAHA*

(Phonetic pronunciation: *aum shreem luhk shm yi nuh muh hu*)

Salutations to Goddess Lakshmi, the goddess of good fortune.

Synchronise your breath with the mantra.

If you prefer you can call to her in your own language, for example:

'Oh Goddess Lakshmi, I honour you as Shakti, I ask for blessings of abundance, generosity, equilibrium and sovereignty. Blessing to you dear One.'

Continue focusing on breath and mantra for as long as you feel comfortable to do so, 10–30 minutes is a nice length of time.

Gradually, release the mantra and the visualisation.

Become aware of your body in contact with the ground once more and take time to externalise your awareness before completing your practice.

Rainbow meditation

This meditation is like having an energetic spring clean and fine tune. Take your time. Refer to the appendix page 159 if you wish for further detail regarding the chakras. In this practice, we use the high vibration of the rainbow within the subtle body. When we rest here, we feel our completeness.

To begin, either lie down or sit in a comfortable posture.

Become aware of the ground supporting you and the sky above.

Bring your awareness to the base of the body, mooladara chakra, located just inside the lower lips. Breathe here.

Here, visualise, sense, or imagine a deep red colour. As you breathe naturally allow this red colour to expand and fill your body.

Allow your awareness to move upward, along the central energy channel (sushumna nadi) to swadithana chakra located between the tail bone and front of pelvis. Breathe here and visualise the colour orange.

As you breathe naturally allow this orange colour to expand and fill your body.

Release awareness of the colour orange at swadithana and move your awareness up to behind the navel, manipur chakra.

Breathing at manipur, here visualise a bright yellow colour. Allow this yellow colour to expand and fill your whole being.

Allow the awareness to ascend to the heart space, anahat chakra. Breathe here and imagine, sense, or visualise a green colour. As you breathe the colour green extends into your whole body.

Release awareness at anahat and come to the throat centra or vishuddi chakra. At vishuddhi, visualise a bright blue colour. Breathe awareness at vishuddhi and visualising the colour blue, allow this blue colour to fill your body.

Allow the awareness to move upwards to the centre of the head. Here at agya chakra visualise the colour indigo. Breathe at agya and become aware of this indigo colour expanding and filling your whole being, every cell absorbed in indigo.

Release this now and allow the awareness to rest at the crown, sahasr-ara. Here visualise the colour violet and white. Visualise this violet-white colour filling your whole being, including the space around the body.

Become aware of all the colours of the rainbow within the body. Feel the vibrational energy of the rainbow. Rest in this frequency.

Become aware of your breath and the solidity of the physical body.

Notice the sounds around you.

Feel the body sitting on the ground, continue to externalise your awareness.

Yoga nidra—Initiation into wise woman circle

For this practice, I suggest you read aloud the script and record it so you can use it when you wish. Read it in a clear voice at a steady pace. Ensure that you won't be interrupted.

Lie in shavasana or a semi-supine position. Allow a little space between your arms and the side of body and space between the ankles. You may like to place a bolster or folded blanket beneath your knees or lower thighs.

Remove any bulky jewellery or glasses.

During the practice I will refer to your *sankalpa*. A sankalpa is your resolve, it is a short positive statement about your life that you will repeat several times during the practice. The seed of the sankalpa is planted in your unconscious, allowing it to flourish without resistance. Choose something that has real value and meaning to you before you begin the practice. A sankalpa is an affirming statement spoken in the present tense, for example: 'I am moving towards fulfilling my soul's purpose.'

Set an intention to remain awake and aware during the practice.

Make any final adjustments to body or clothing. Allow the body to become still, only move if there is pain or significant discomfort.

Become aware of the connection between body and ground. All the parts of the body in connection with the body and ground. The feet, legs, buttocks, back, all the parts of the back, hands and arms, and the back of the head.

With every breath allow the body to become more relaxed and have a sense of letting go into the earth, knowing that She is supporting you and there is nothing for you to do but listen to the instructions.

Silently repeat your sankalpa, the positive affirming statement about your life. Repeat it with deep faith and conviction.

The next part of the practice is the rotation of awareness around the body. Follow my voice and as each part of the body is named, bring your awareness to that body part and mentally repeat the name of that part of the body.

Awareness to right hand ... right hand thumb ... second finger ... third finger ... fourth finger ... fifth finger ... palm of hand ... back of hand ... wrist ... forearm ... elbow ... upper arm ... right shoulder ... armpit ... side of body ... waist ... hip ... thigh ... knee ... back of knee ... shin ... calf ... heel ... top of right foot ... sole of foot ... big toe ... second toe ... third toe ... fourth toe ... fifth toe ...

Awareness now to left hand ... left hand thumb ... second finger ... third finger ... fourth finger ... fifth finger ... palm of hand ... back of hand ... wrist ... forearm ... elbow ... upper arm ... left shoulder ... armpit ... side of body ... waist ... hip ... thigh ... knee ... back of knee ... shin ... calf ... heel ... top of left foot ... sole of foot ... big toe ... second toe ... third toe ... fourth toe ... fifth toe ...

Awareness to right buttock ... left buttock ... lower back ... middle back ... upper back ... the whole of the back ... the spinal column ... the whole of the back ... back of neck ... back of head ... top of head ... forehead ... right temple ... left temple ... right ear ... left ear ... right eyebrow ... left eyebrow ... the space between the eyebrows ... right eye ... left eye ... right cheek ... left cheek ... right nostril ... left nostril ... tip of nose ... upper lip ... lower lip ... space where lips meet ... tongue ... teeth ... chin ... jaw ... throat ... right collar bone ... left collar bone ... right breast ... left breast ... centre of the chest ... upper abdomen ... lower abdomen ... navel ... the womb space ... the elimination organs ...

The whole of the right side of body ... whole of left side of body ... right and left side of body together ... the front of body ... back of body ... front and back of the body together ... the whole of the body ... awareness of the whole of the body, whole body awareness.

Become aware now of your breath ... the body breathing in and body breathing out ... feel the sensation of breath on your nostrils, sensation of breath ... in the upper lungs ... lower lungs ... abdomen ... awareness of abdomen expanding with the inhalation and contracting with exhalation ... become aware of the body breathing ... continue being aware of the natural breath for several minutes.

Become aware of the sensation of heaviness ... allow the body to feel heavy. Surrender the whole body to the sensation of heaviness ...

heaviness in the feet ... legs ... hips ... back ... arms ... and hands ... the whole torso feeling so, so heavy ... the head, and skull so heavy you can barely lift it ... the whole body feeling heavier and heavier, as if made of stone ... a dead weight ... a heavy, heavy body ... release the sensation of heaviness in the body now ... fully let go of the sensation of a heavy body.

Allow yourself to experience the sensation now of a light body ... the whole body feeling weightless and light ... lightness in the fingers and toes, feet and hands ... the arms and legs, so light they could lift off the ground ... weightless body ... torso feeling so, so light and the head and skull as light as a feather. Allow yourself to fully experience the sensation of a light body. Release the sensation of lightness in the body now ... fully let go of the sensation of a weightless body.

Bring your awareness to your eyebrow centre, the activation point for agya chakra ... allow yourself to breath here ... inhale into eyebrow centre ... exhale from eyebrow centre. Continue this for several breaths.

Bring the awareness to the dark space behind the eyes, the place of visions and dreams. Create some images, use your imagination, visualisation, or sense them. Imagine you are walking along in nature ... It is dusk and the light is beginning to fade ... there is enough light for you to follow the path and you notice plants on either side of the path and hear birds preparing for the night ... you continue along the path as it winds and bends, the plants become shrubs and trees. You reach a woodland, it is dark now ... you see a flicker of light through the undergrowth ... you walk towards it, there you see a fire burning bright, around it is a circle of women ... they are swaying and humming ... you have a feeling that you have been here before ... one of the women sees you, smiles, and beckons you to join them, you step into the circle and are greeted as an old friend ... as you take your place in the circle of women you become aware of a connection with the fire at the centre and also the circle of women ... a woman comes and stands before you, she looks deep into your eyes and holds out a golden goblet towards you inviting you to drink pure spring water ... you take the golden goblet and bring it to your lips, knowing that as you do so you are being initiated into this wise woman circle ... you drink deeply, feeling a deep ancient thirst being quenched ... you look around the circle and all the women are welcoming you, their eyes sparkling with love and acceptance ... the circle beginning to sway and move as one ... you sing and dance with the women. The wood is dark now and the fire begins to burn low ... it is time to leave the circle ... you offer your gratitude and take your leave, knowing that you can return at any time and reconnect with this circle ... an owl hoots three times ... you make your way back along the path ...

Let go of this visualisation now ... bring the awareness to the heart space ... It is time for you to repeat your sankalpa once again, repeating it several times to yourself with faith and conviction that it is manifesting in your life ... release your sankalpa now ... become aware of your whole body, the outline and physicality of your body ... know that the yoga nidra will soon be coming to an end ... become aware of the contact between floor and feet ... legs ... contact between the back and the ground ... the ground making contact with the arms and hands ... and the back of the head ... all the points of contact between body and ground ... become aware of the room that you are in ... noticing the body breathing and allow a couple of deeper breaths ... now that the yoga nidra is concluding ... continue to externalise your awareness ... gently allow the head to roll to one side then the other ... bring gentle movement to fingers and toes ... bring the knees up to the chest and give yourself a hug ... stretch and yawn ... when you are ready you can sit up ... take your time.

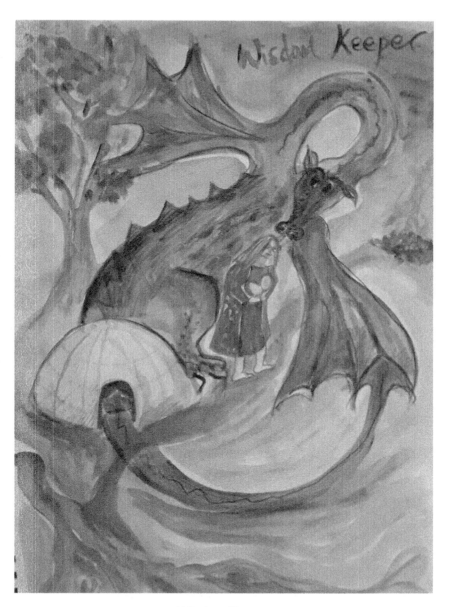

Wisdom Keeper

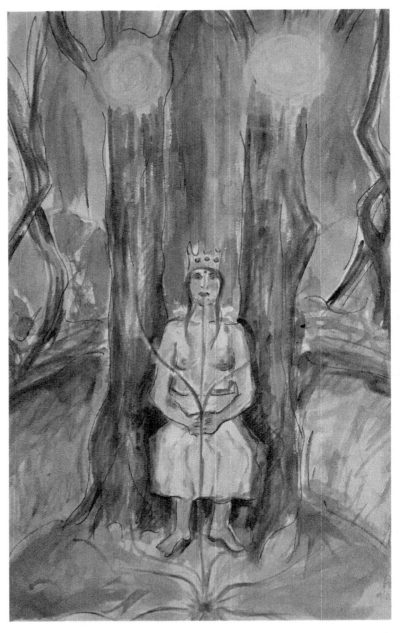

Sovereignty

CHAPTER 9

Wise Woman Celebration

Choosing the right time to celebrate your menopausal rite of passage is important. This means *your* right time and not someone else's. A woman on a sacred feminine retreat shared that her girlfriends had kindly organised a 'becoming crone' celebration for her on her fiftieth birthday. However, she was still bleeding and finding her way through perimenopause, she was not ready to celebrate this initiation but did not want to hurt her friends' feelings.

You may wish to wait until your second Saturn Return at around age fifty-nine. The first being around age twenty-nine. From an astrological perspective, this is where you have completed that phase of maturation, the old is released and we step into a new cycle. During early perimenopause I had imagined inviting a few friends to witness a ceremony, however, when I turned inwards to feel into if this felt right, it didn't—the inward facing aspect of the journey means that to celebrate and be witnessed may not feel right for some time. The Saturn Return is referred to as the *second quest* or pushing us to resolve anything before our third act of life. This is often described as needing focus, clarity, and stamina just as we experience in our menopause initiation.

This is a time to embrace your inner witch. You may feel that you are not yet crone, that you feel more akin to the priestess, wise woman, or matriarch. Be authentic and real about where you are and find the language that honours that as best as you can during your celebration.

Create your ceremony in a way that feels right for you. You may wish to consider who you want to be there, perhaps women that have supported or inspired you, perhaps different ages of women, do you want men there, your partner? Consider season, time of day, place, get it just right. Like any celebration, is there particular food or drink, for example mead and chocolate cake! Do you want guests to wear something, what do you want to wear? During the rite of passage of menarche increasingly many young women are gifted with sensitive elders to guide and honour them. One of the ways a mother shared was that she had given her daughter a red blanket to use during her bleed, this not only brought her comfort but also communicated to the rest of the family where she was in her cycle. Similarly, you may wish to consider in what ways you can mark this transition. I, for example, have a necklace that I wear when I am resonating strongly with my crone and/or Goddess Kali energy. It helps me to remember who I am and accept this expression of myself with honour.

Below are two ceremony suggestions. Be creative and find your own that encompasses and expresses who you are and the journey you have been on.

Celebration Ceremony: reflecting and looking forward

This is based on a linear time thread and can be beautiful witnessed by a group of friends who you feel safe with and wish to celebrate with.

Place a red cord, rope or length of material across a room or space in nature. Stand at one end of the space, the cord dividing it horizontally. The starting place corresponds with the beginning of your journey. You may wish to start at birth or from when you began your bleed. If you haven't previously honoured your menses and practised conscious menstruation this may be particularly poignant.

Take your time to recall any feelings, significant memories about place, time, people, and experience. When ready, begin to take a step forward, moving through your life with each step. Some parts may be quicker than others, you may wish to pause and linger, recalling points in your life journey.

Speak aloud anything you wish to be witnessed. Allow the body to take any movement or shape to help embody your journey.

The red cord symbolises the end of your bleeding. As you arrive here, look back on your journey so far. When ready step over the cord, knowing that this is you stepping forward into a new life phase, the time of wise woman, moving into crone. See the space before you, the unshaped, spacious, blank canvas of what lies before you. Feel the anticipation and excitement of a new beginning.

Invite your witnesses to clap, bang drums and rattles, and cheer as you step over the initiation threshold.

Celebration Ceremony—circle of women

This is a nice ceremony to do with friends that have known you a while as it supports you in acknowledging that you have changed and helps them recognise this as well as validating it to yourself.

You may like to hold this ceremony in nature, or in a place that has been made beautifully befitting. You will need several lengths of ribbon, material, or cord.

Stand at the centre of the circle of friends. One by one they hold a thread and tie the other end to you, using clothing or a specific made belt or garment. As they do this, the friends say something about you and as they do so they wrap the thread around you. For example, 'Jane has courage and speaks her truth', 'Jane is a great mother'. When all the threads are tied and words spoken, you wriggle and break free from the cocoon of threads, symbolic of your transformation and metamorphosis of your menopause passage.

When free you speak your new truth, defining youself in any way you choose, e.g. 'I have the freedom to follow my own energy', 'I am ready to share what I have learnt'. The witnessing circle listen and can make sounds to acknowledge what has been said, for example, 'a new beginning, a new way, yes!'

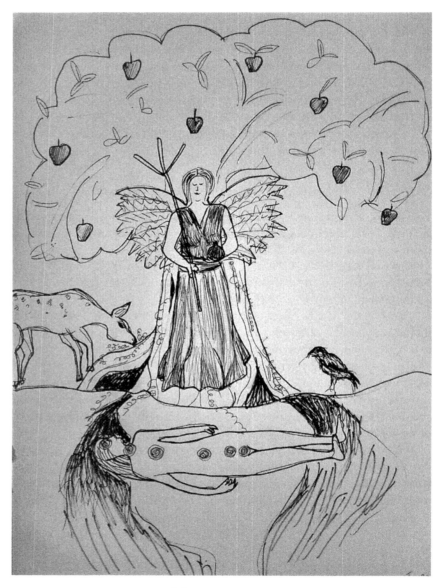

Celebration Ceremony

CHAPTER 10

Welcome Relief from Menopause Experiences

During your menopause there are many different experiences that you may have, and this list is not exhaustive. As I have previously said, every woman is unique and this will include the different physical, mental, emotional, and energetic symptoms she will have. As we cease to release eggs our hormone levels change, particularly through a lowering of estrogen and progesterone (menopausematters.co.uk). I have put some of these experiences into the chart below so that you can refer easily to a different way of thinking about it which can be helpful when in the midst of it. Remember that 'energy flows where awareness goes', so be aware of where your focus is and what you are reinforcing.

I have offered prompts to perspective, practice, holistic therapies, and occasionally herbs—but I am not a trained herbalist and mention only those that I or women I know have found helpful. Sage, Red Clover, and Lemon Balm are widely available and can easily be collected for tea—they offer support for a wide range of experiences and are excellent menopause medicine. Please do consult a local herbalist for further guidance. When foraging and collecting herbs it is interesting to feel into which plant is calling you. When picking take a moment to connect with the plant and ask if you may take, giving thanks if you do.

Many women find exercise helpful both to keep energy flowing in the body with strength and flexibility, and to help keep the mind in a good space. If you are unable to resonate with the suggestions or they irritate you, then follow your own thread that will soothe you. Use whatever it takes, this may include delight in foraging, use of gemstones, homeopathy, and body treatments. Think holistic and outside your usual terrain. This may also include making the decision to take hormone replacement therapy. As with many of the experiences or symptoms, practices that support acceptance such as meditation are useful.

One way to perceive any physical symptom is as stagnant or blocked energy. When we hold our experiences like this, we also hold the knowing that they can change, they are not set or chronic or forever. This simple shift in perspective can soften our mindset around the experience. You may find it helpful to work from both a physical and energetic perspective. You may also wish to include increased discipline in choosing your thoughts and feelings, allowing those that may be related to be changed. These symptoms and experiences can continue for several years, perhaps a decade, following the year after our last bleed.

I know as much as anyone that it is one thing saying it and another doing it. When we are in menopause, as in our autumn or winter of our moon cycle, the time when we should care more for ourselves is often also the time when we can't be bothered and don't care. However, as Myra Lewin (2017) helpfully says, just move a little in the direction that you wish to go. If you turn in the opposite direction, just say 'oops' and re-adjust and begin again. These suggestions are from things that I have found helpful or know other women who have. The best advice is from yourself. Remember that although you may wish to navigate your menopause naturally, if you don't that's ok too. A decision to use hormone replacement therapy from a place of awareness and acceptance can sometimes be the best decision for yourself.

Sometimes it can help just to do something totally different to usual. This can shake something free, allow a space, a new space for the metamorphosis to take shape, it can bring insights. I have always been resistant to sport, and yet during menopause I felt a whisper to run. When I finally conceded I found it made me feel alive and as my friend said you have to propel yourself forward. I also had a memory recall of running cross country as a young teenager at school. The jog directly linked, or jogged me, to recall my menarche initiation. When we do something outside our usual parameter, whether that's smoking a cigarette, sky diving, staying in bed until midday, or naked wild swimming, our system is rewiring and recalibrating. We are aligning with our higher self's wish for expansion and growth.

Food

One of the main things we can do to support ourselves during this time is to use food skillfully. There is much conflicting advice about food, so it really is a time for you to follow what makes sense to you and your body. If you're reading this book, you are probably well aware that to have a good, varied diet of fresh produce will serve you well.

Some women have had a complex journey with their relationship to food, including dieting to lose weight, erratic or emotional eating and specific diets to improve health. I believe that the most important thing is to regard food with appreciation and pleasure. If we cook and eat with guilt and anxiety, we are also ingesting those vibrations which will not nourish us.

I will share a few thoughts from an ayurvedic perspective, as I believe this ancient tradition supports the endocrine system in a holistic way. As I described in the Introduction, in Ayurveda, menopause is a time of increased vata and often vata dosha imbalance. To balance vata we need to eat nourishing, augmenting foods. This can include root vegetables such as sweet potato, carrot, and beetroot. Grains such as short grain brown rice, white basmati, barley and wheat also help. If we refer to the elements, we can see that if we have too much air element, we can balance this by introducing more foods related to the element of earth.

It can also help to approach our meals as the priestess would. Eating as a sacred act, taking time and giving it our full awareness. Taking time to become calm and connected to our body before we eat can support digestion. Chewing our food thoroughly, ideally to mush, also helps our bodies digest and extract the nutrients from our food, our saliva being the start of the digestive process.

We need good oils such as ghee (clarified butter), olive oil, and coconut oil. Ghee is particularly helpful in nourishing our mind and body. It can lubricate joints, soften our edges and maintain healthy hair and skin. It is satisfying and easy to make, see Hale Pule in Further Resources, page 171 for guidance on how to make ghee.

There are many excellent books about Ayurveda, so I will not duplicate here. The main thing is to keep the fire in the gut *agni* strong and to reduce vata. It is also helpful to remember this guideline:

"Like attracts like and the opposite brings balance." (Lewin, 2017)

The suggestions below all support this. They are not complicated or expensive, just common sense, traditional things that can make a big difference to how we feel. We don't want to set up resistance by feeling that they are *shoulds*. Simply hold these guidelines loosely and use them when it feels aligned to your own energy and truth.

Food and Eating Habits to Support You

Do not drink large amounts of liquid immediately before, after, or with your meal.

Relax and chew thoroughly in a calm environment.

Drink herbal teas throughout the day or warm water. Ginger tea is excellent to stimulate digestion.

Eat nourishing heavier foods, avoid lots of light crisp foods, such as salad and crackers.

Avoid overeating, eat what you can hold in your two hands.

Avoid snacking as this will weaken your digestive fire.

Reduce caffeine.

Reduce refined sugar.

Reduce alcohol.

Eat simply but with good quality ingredients.

Enjoy your food, knowing it is nourishing, healing, and sustaining you.

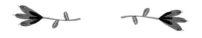

Menopause Experiences and Welcome Relief
Achey Bones

As our hormones change, we can experience changes in our bone density. The menopause is associated with osteoporosis. Weight bearing exercises are often suggested and these may help. As we grow into our crone years, we are experiencing growing pains. These are natural and communicate to us that we are in a process of change and initiation.

Bone breathing

Lie on the floor. Become aware of the ground beneath you and the earth supporting you.

Begin to allow the body to soften and relax.

Allow gravity to let the body sink into the earth.

Become aware of your breath, your natural breath. As you inhale imagine, sense, or visualise breathing in energy from the earth. As you exhale, with your will and intention move this energy to your bones.

With each breath allow this earth energy to nourish your skeleton.

Ancestral ritual

Our bones connect us to our ancestors. See Chapter 3, 'My Wild Indigenous Body', page 42.

Herbal support

Horsetail and Nettle tea are both packed full of minerals that support bone health and make a potent tea blend.

Erratic Bleeding

Erratic bleeding can begin in our forties and can signal a need for increased self-care. Balance vata dosha and the air element in the body. If you are a woman who has relied upon the regularity of your bleed, this may be disorientating and anxiety provoking. Adjust to make it easier, this may mean wearing a pad in addition to your moon cup and carrying spare clothes in your car if you fear flooding.

Oiling the body

The ayurvedic practice of *abyanga* helps to nourish the body and is calming to the nervous system and reduces vata dosha or excess air element. This is a practice that you can do daily or occasionally.

Warm a little sesame or olive oil by standing the cup of oil in a bowl of hot water. Take your time with this practice, being aware of the sensation and luxuriate in the self-care.

Apply the oil to the skin using long, slow, firm touch. Move from the middle body including hips, buttocks and waist and then move down the legs. At the joints, the knees, ankles and hips you can apply the oil in a circular motion.

Work along the sides of the body, around the navel (clockwise, once or twice), on the lower back. Reaching as much of the back as possible.

Circle the shoulders, elbows and wrists and move down the arms, applying oil to the hands and fingers. Continue by applying oil to the breasts in circular motions and armpits.

Apply the oil to the neck, shoulders and gently to the face. Use the fingertips to gently tap and then pinch along the eyebrows and jaw line. Oil can be applied to the scalp if you wish.

If possible, lie down on an old towel, making sure you are warm enough and rest, allowing the oil to absorb into the tissues of the body for 10–20 minutes. You can then have a warm shower, without using products.

(It is a good idea to pour a kettle of boiling water down the shower drain after you have finished your practice to prevent any issues with the drainage.)

In Ayurveda, the practice of oiling the body can be helpful in calming the mind and nervous system.

Eat nourishing foods

Eat warm, nourishing foods such as root vegetables.

Herbal support

Agnus Castus tincture, Motherwort, Mugwort and Lady's Mantle, the leaves of which can be found in most gardens and can be made into tea, help regulate and maintain rhythm with the moon cycle particularly during perimenopause and help moderate excessive bleeding (consult a herbalist.)

Journey to your womb

You may like to use a shamanic drum beat or recording for this practice.

Hold your intention to journey into your womb space, repeat your intention several times to yourself.

Allow your awareness to move into your womb space. See what emerges, ask to meet a guide. Have a conversation, ask what is going on, what is needed at this time.

Remain open and receptive to what may arise such as a healing or guidance; what are you being shown?

If it appears that nothing much is happening or you feel stuck, repeat your intention and rest your awareness in the womb space.

Return with the call of the drum, either at a time set at the beginning of your journey or at a time when your awareness is ready to shift.

Journal and reflect upon your experience. Remember that everything in your experience of the journey is part of your answer, guidance, and healing.

Yoni Soreness

The lining of the vagina can become thinner and sensitive which can make love-making challenging. Consider approaches discussed in Chapter 7, 'The Priestess is in the Temple', page 81. You may wish to experiment with a natural lubricant such as saliva, coconut oil, or aloe vera gel. Give your yoni love, use self-massage to nourish her and increase blood flow and pranic energy. You may wish to explore using a jade egg. Breast massage may also support the yoni. Once when I was talking to a friend about the positive aspects of menopause, she snarled at me, 'it's not very empowering when your vagina collapses', and of course she is right, atrophy is upsetting and may include processing emotions such as sadness and anger.

Nourishment from the earth

This practice is based upon the yogic *moola bandha* and the Lyceum practice of *star sipping*.

Sit in a comfortable meditation posture. Relax the mouth and the jaw. Allow the body to be relaxed but maintaining length and space through the spine.

Become aware of the contact between the base of the body and the ground. Awareness of your solid, stable base. Bring the awareness to the mooladhara chakra, located inside the yoni towards your cervix.

Allow your awareness to descend downwards, through the ground from the base of the body. Moving through layers of soil, and rock, moving towards the centre of the earth. Use your imagination and intention. At the centre of the earth star is a ball of energy and light.

As you inhale, allow your awareness to draw up some of this energy into the womb space. As you inhale, gently contract the muscles of the vagina or moola bandha. This is a subtle movement.

As you exhale, release. Continue inhaling, bringing the energy up into the body's alchemical vessel, bringing nourishment, vitality, and energy. Ensure that you are not straining breath or yoni muscles, fully relax as you exhale.

Pause as you wish. When you are ready, let go of the awareness of the earth star, moola bandha, and awareness at mooladhara. Become aware of the effects of your practice.

Externalise your awareness.

This practice can also be done with small, short contractions, like small sips of energy. As the yoni muscles pulse, keep the breath slow and deep.

Yoni circular breath

See Chapter 2, page 27 and adapt it by using the energy of natural things that support juiciness, such as honey or oil in your practice.

Nourishing breath

Either lying down or sitting in a comfortable meditation posture.

Inhale deeply down the front of your body, feeling the breath fill the genitals, bringing energy into the yoni and lower mouth. With the exhalation, circulate the breath up the spinal column. Continue in this way.

As you inhale you may wish to synchronise with the breath the thought, 'I inhale nourishing energy to my yoni', as you exhale 'I release and surrender, offering my unique gifts to the world.'

Brain Fog

Hold gratitude and the knowing that the right and left brain are being rebalanced and recalibrated at this time. This rebalancing is supporting you in developing increased intuitive faculties. When we experience poor memory and brain fog, we have more present moment awareness. This is hugely sought after in many spiritual traditions, so regard it as a blessing. Where possible reduce responsibilities. Notice how when people have expectations about how you should think and what you should retain, they are usually coming from a learnt left brain, masculine perspective. Remind yourself that you are in a different process with different priorities at this time of growth.

Herbal support

Have a sprig of Rosemary with you to sniff or use essential oil to help stimulate memory and cognitive function.

Red Clover tincture or tea is an excellent menopause all-rounder. It can help manage the hormone changes that can lead to lack of mental clarity and brain fog. Consult a herbalist.

Balancing both

See practices described in Chapter 7, 'The Priestess is in the House', such as nadi shodhana, to balance left and right brain and body.

Agya chakra

See meditation practice 'Agya awakening' described in Chapter 6, page 78. This will help bring clarity and more confidence in your second sight.

Achey Muscles

As with achey bones our muscles ache because we are in a process of metamorphosis. Our muscles can also hold stress and trauma. We are invited to face, explore, and release these in our underworld journey and Chiron Return.

Oiling your body

Using oil such as olive or sesame oil on the skin can help nourish and relax muscles.

Warm a little oil by standing the cup of oil in a bowl of hot water. Take your time with this practice, being aware of the sensation and luxuriate in the self-care.

Apply the oil to the skin using long, slow, firm touch. Move from the middle body including hips, buttocks and waist and then move down the legs. At the joints, the knees, ankles and hips you can apply the oil in a circular motion.

Work along the sides of the body, around the navel (clockwise, once or twice), on the lower back. Reaching as much of the back as possible.

Circle the shoulders, elbows and wrists and move down the arms, applying oil to the hands and fingers. Continue by applying oil to the breasts in circular motions and armpits.

Apply the oil to the neck, shoulders and gently to the face. Use the fingertips to gently tap and then pinch along the eyebrows and jaw line. Oil can be applied to the scalp if you wish.

If possible, lie down on an old towel, making sure you are warm enough and rest, allowing the oil to absorb into the tissues of the body for 10–20 minutes. You can then have a warm shower, without using products.

(It is a good idea to pour a kettle of boiling water down the shower drain after you have finished your practice to prevent any issues with the drainage.)

In Ayurveda, the practice of oiling the body can be helpful in calming the mind and nervous system.

Internal oiling

Use ghee in cooking, ideally a spoonful in every meal, this helps lubricate the body and eases achey muscles and joints. It is easy to make and helps keep the body deeply nourished and lubricated. (see Further Resources page 171, Hale Pule).

Intuitive movement

As you move begin to feel into how your body wishes to move. There may be a particular focal point such as your leg or neck. How does this body part want to move, lead and express itself? Allow the body to lead.

Shaking

This can help release any habitual holding or tension in the body and bring increased blood to the muscles. See Chapter 1, page 12 for more guidance about this practice.

Herbal support

Using a magnesium spray or taking it orally can help in reducing muscle pain, discomfort, and inflammation. Meadowsweet taken as a herbal tea can also ease discomfort and inflammation.

Anxiety

Having an awareness of the hormonal changes that are occurring can help. Where possible reduce your responsibilities. Focus on calming and supporting your adrenal system. Anxiety signals that we are realigning to our inner being. You may also be absorbing other disturbances from individuals and the collective. Know that you are becoming more sensitive to energies. Keep releasing into the earth and explore surrounding yourself with protective light.

Breath awareness

Lie in the dark.

Place one hand on your womb space and the other on your heart. Or, if you prefer have your arms by the sides of your body.

Bring your awareness to your natural breath. Notice the movement in the abdomen … the sensations at the nostrils.

When the mind wanders just gently bring it back to the breath and sensations.

Continue in this way for 5–20 minutes.

Reduce stimulation

Reduce electronic use, including phone, Wi-Fi, computer, and electricity.

Consciously take some time to be in silence.

Yoga nidra

The practice of yoga nidra can assist in relaxing the mind and body. It moves us into theta brain wave state and para-sympathetic nervous system. See Chapter 1, page 8, Chapter 4, page 55 and Chapter 8, page 109 for the yoga nidra scripts or listen to recordings via website.

Walk barefoot

Set aside some time in nature and walk barefoot.

You may like to focus and do a meditation walk, having awareness on the different parts of the foot as they come into contact
with the earth.

Or you may like to walk easefully and naturally, letting your feet
lead.

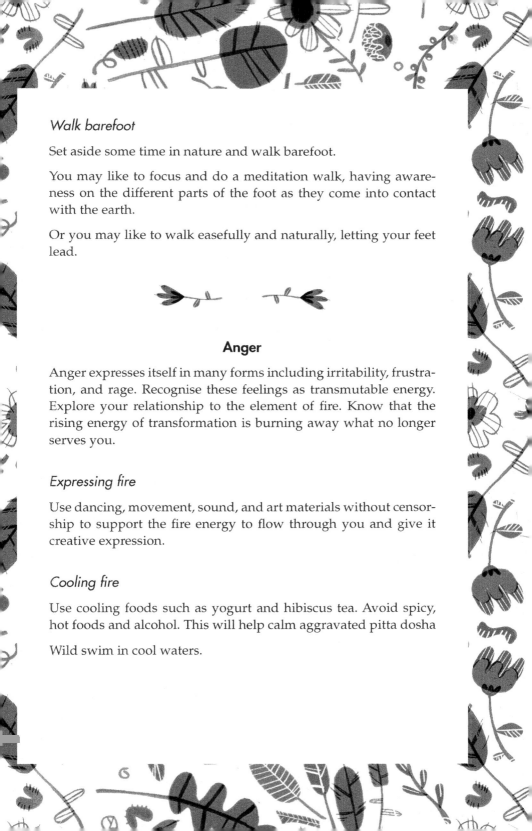

Anger

Anger expresses itself in many forms including irritability, frustra-
tion, and rage. Recognise these feelings as transmutable energy.
Explore your relationship to the element of fire. Know that the
rising energy of transformation is burning away what no longer
serves you.

Expressing fire

Use dancing, movement, sound, and art materials without censorship to support the fire energy to flow through you and give it
creative expression.

Cooling fire

Use cooling foods such as yogurt and hibiscus tea. Avoid spicy,
hot foods and alcohol. This will help calm aggravated pitta dosha

Wild swim in cool waters.

Fire ritual

Having a fire ritual gives a focused intention and space for strong emotions such as anger. Fire helps transform energy. For further details of fire practices that you may wish to adapt see Chapter 1, page 13, and Chapter 3, page 42.

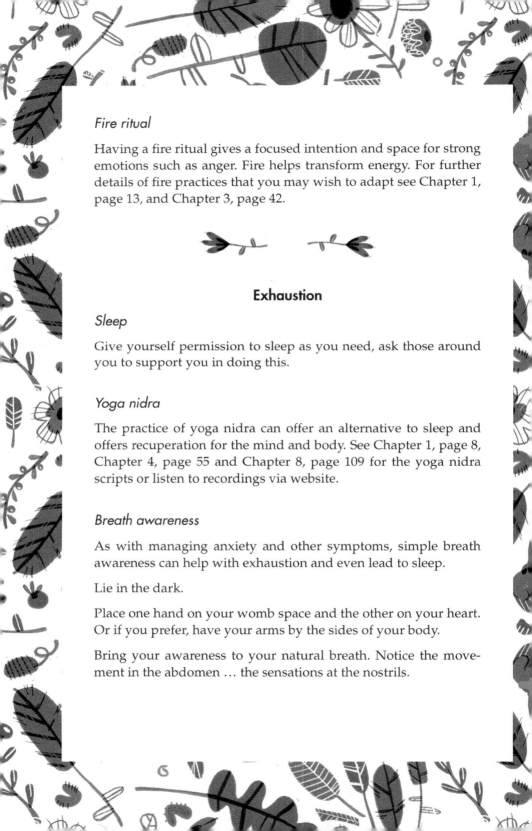

Exhaustion

Sleep

Give yourself permission to sleep as you need, ask those around you to support you in doing this.

Yoga nidra

The practice of yoga nidra can offer an alternative to sleep and offers recuperation for the mind and body. See Chapter 1, page 8, Chapter 4, page 55 and Chapter 8, page 109 for the yoga nidra scripts or listen to recordings via website.

Breath awareness

As with managing anxiety and other symptoms, simple breath awareness can help with exhaustion and even lead to sleep.

Lie in the dark.

Place one hand on your womb space and the other on your heart. Or if you prefer, have your arms by the sides of your body.

Bring your awareness to your natural breath. Notice the movement in the abdomen … the sensations at the nostrils.

When the mind wanders just gently bring it back to the breath and sensations.

Continue in this way for 5–20 minutes.

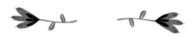

Lack of Enthusiasm

Trust that this will change. Know that you are gaining clarity about who you are and what your preferences are and what you desire. Lack of enthusiasm can be a call to explore and experiment new terrain.

Seek out something different—watch a film you wouldn't usually watch, go to the circus, absail, trampoline, lie in a pit covered in leaves, go to a charity shop and buy clothes you would never usually consider, enjoy exploring different personas. Allow the experience to touch you within in a new way, allow it to shift your awareness or gain more clarity regarding your preferences.

Cultivate present moment awareness

Use your senses to bring as much awareness as possible to the present moment. Look at a flower, an insect, the touch of clothes on skin, the smell of the rain.

You may also like to imagine that as you observe these things, they are observing you. You may also like to imagine or sense that they are desiring and inviting a relationship and dialogue. Explore this experience.

Appreciation

At the end of the day take a few moments to recall three things that you were grateful for in your day.

This could be an interaction you had, something you saw or just that your body breathed.

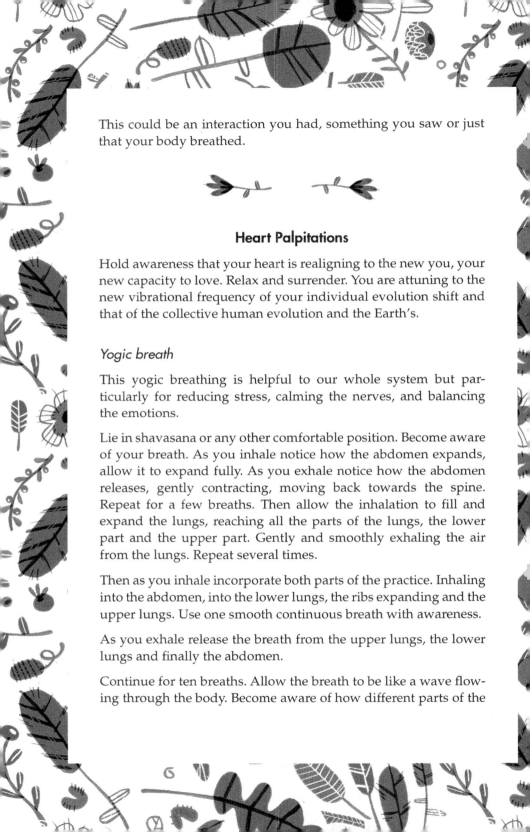

Heart Palpitations

Hold awareness that your heart is realigning to the new you, your new capacity to love. Relax and surrender. You are attuning to the new vibrational frequency of your individual evolution shift and that of the collective human evolution and the Earth's.

Yogic breath

This yogic breathing is helpful to our whole system but particularly for reducing stress, calming the nerves, and balancing the emotions.

Lie in shavasana or any other comfortable position. Become aware of your breath. As you inhale notice how the abdomen expands, allow it to expand fully. As you exhale notice how the abdomen releases, gently contracting, moving back towards the spine. Repeat for a few breaths. Then allow the inhalation to fill and expand the lungs, reaching all the parts of the lungs, the lower part and the upper part. Gently and smoothly exhaling the air from the lungs. Repeat several times.

Then as you inhale incorporate both parts of the practice. Inhaling into the abdomen, into the lower lungs, the ribs expanding and the upper lungs. Use one smooth continuous breath with awareness.

As you exhale release the breath from the upper lungs, the lower lungs and finally the abdomen.

Continue for ten breaths. Allow the breath to be like a wave flowing through the body. Become aware of how different parts of the body are affected, even when relaxed, including the diaphragm and the sensation in the throat.

Yoga nidra

The practice of yoga nidra can shift our nervous system into a para-sympathetic state which allows us to relax. This will support the heart finding its natural rhythm again. See Chapter 1, page 8, Chapter 4, page 55 and Chapter 8, page 109 for the yoga nidra scripts or listen to recordings via website.

Mary Magdalene rose meditation

Come into a comfortable sitting or lying posture. Release any tension in the body by bringing the awareness to each body part or area and consciously releasing.

Feel held and supported by the ground.

If you wish you can begin the meditation by asking Mary Magdalene to be present. By invoking Mary Magdalene we draw upon the Divine Feminine and all that she embodies.

Bring your awareness to the heart space. Visualise, sense, or imagine breathing from the heart space. Inhaling and exhaling naturally and simply.

Imagine a rose, a pale pink rose at the heart space.

As you inhale allow the petals of this rose to gently expand. As you exhale allow the petals to soften and gently contract.

Imagine the rose diffusing the light of the rose colour, pale pink expanding into the body space with the exhalation.

As you continue with your breath and awareness at the heart space and the rose, become aware of the scent of the rose.

As you inhale allow the scent of the rose to fill the heart space.

As you exhale allow the scent to expand and fill the body.

Allow the body and heart space to be like a soft cocoon, gently moving with the breath, softly expanding with the rose-coloured light and the scent of the rose. Gently contracting, wave after wave of breath, light and perfumed scent of rose.

Continue in this way for 5–20 minutes.

When ready, release the awareness of the rose and its light and scent.

Become aware of the skin boundary of the body and the solidity of the body.

If it feels right to you, offer your gratitude to Mary Magdalene.

Continue to externalise your awareness. Appreciate the subtle effects of your practice.

Herbal support

Motherwort tea and hawthorn berries crushed as tea or tincture can offer support to the heart.

Sciatica

This experience encourages you to work with your energy flow between your earth and sky connection. Do you feel held between the sky and earth? Develop your connection to rooting down-wards and also lifting upwards into spaciousness.

Shaking

This can help release any habitual holding or tension in the body and bring increased blood to the muscles. Make sure you are con-necting to the earth through your feet, aware of your roots and your lower body supported by the earth's energy. See Chapter 1, page 12 for more guidance about this practice.

Releasing sciatica

Lying on your back with your knees bent and feet hip width apart, the soles of the feet on the ground.

Slowly, clench the buttocks and then release.

Repeat this 10–30 times.

(Egoscue, 2022)

Jogging

Some women find walking or jogging helpful during menopause, especially for sciatica. This may not be for everyone, so as always do what feels right for you. Make sure you look after knees and have good supportive footwear, unless barefoot.

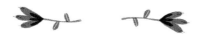

Hot Flush

During menopause the kundalini is rising. The spiritual fire of initiation and transformation is burning off the old 'dross'. Relax and let the fire burn what no longer serves you. If need be use these cooling practices for relief.

Sheetali

Sheetali is a pranayama practice also known as cooling breath and has a soothing effect.

Sit comfortably in meditation posture. Close eyes and relax. Extend the tongue outside the mouth without straining. Roll the sides of the tongue inward, to create a roll or tube. Inhale long and deep through the tongue. Bring the tongue in and exhale through the nose.

Continue for several rounds until you feel cool (approx. 10–30).

Sheetkari

This is also known as the hissing breath, like sheetali pranayama it is cooling, although not suitable if you have sensitive teeth.

Sit comfortably in meditation posture. Close eyes and relax.

Bring the teeth lightly together, the lips separated. Inhale slowly through the teeth, allowing a hissing sound. Close the mouth. Exhale through the nose.

Continue for several rounds until you feel cool (approx. 10–30).

Circular yoni breath

For guidance about this practice see Chapter 2, page 27 and adapt it by using the energy of natural things that are cooling such as a cool stream, a cool breeze or another cooling aspect of nature.

Herbal support

Red Clover and Hibiscus both have cooling properties and can be used as a tincture or tea. Garden Sage can also help.

Night Sweats

During initiation we experience a purification process. Alchemically, the crucible is being heated and this causes heat and moisture. See yourself as this alchemical vessel.

Sacred fire

Have a fire with intention and give the element of fire—associated with the heat—an outlet. See Chapter 1, page 13 and adapt it for releasing the heat within.

Being in nature

Barefoot, naked, any time of the night, allow yourself to be part of nature, feel the elements and yourself as the elements. If the moon is waxing, breathe in her cool qualities through your skin, bathe in her silvery, cool light. If you are unable to go outside, do this practice through an open window.

Yoga nidra

The practice of yoga nidra can help balance hormones and offers recuperation for the mind and body. See Chapter 1, page 8, Chapter 4, page 55, and Chapter 8, page 109 for the yoga nidra scripts or listen to recordings via website.

Herbal support

Cooling Hibiscus tea can help with night sweats and soothing Chamomile or Sage may also help relieve your experience. Avoid or reduce caffeinated drinks and alcohol.

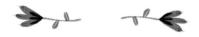

Depression

During menopause you are realigning to follow your own energy and prompts from Source rather than external expectations and roles that you no longer resonate with. Letting go of the old can be emotionally challenging and include grief and depression.

Depression can also be masking unexpressed anger so be honest with yourself and expansive in your inner explorations.

Invoking Goddess Durga

Calling upon our allies that bring comfort and/or determination and resolution to move through depression can be supporting. See meditation practice Chapter 5, page 68.

Circular yoni breath

See Chapter 2, page 27, practise with a yellow flower such as St John's Wort (*Hypericum perforatum*); this flower is commonly known to relieve depression.

Shaking

The practice of shaking can release any stuck emotions; often when we feel depressed there are other emotions such as anger residing beneath. Bringing movement into the body literally shakes up the dominant vibration we are holding. See Chapter 1, page 12.

Dance

Either with music or without, allow yourself to dance freely. Explore in ways that are unfamiliar.

Allow your dance to be authentic. Use the floor and walls to support you, dance with different parts of your body leading, dance with your shadow.

Poor Sleep

We can often find ourselves in a hypervigilant state during the early hours. As our endocrine and nervous system changes and we seek to adapt, we can experience a fight-or-flight response in the early morning as well as erratic sleep. This can be a good time to make the most of the time and to do some gentle practices that will support you through your day even with little sleep.

Mantra repetition

Silently or aloud recite the mantra OM (*AUM*).

Or …

See Chapter 8, page 107 for the Goddess Lakshmi mantra.

See Chapter 3, page 42 for the Goddess Kali mantra.

See Chapter 5, page 68 for the Goddess Durga mantra.

Moonlight breath

If the moon is visible, breathe in her nourishing qualities through your skin, bathe in her silvery, cool light.

If you are unable to go outside do this practice through an open window.

Yoga nidra

The practice of yoga nidra is excellent in calming the nervous system and offers deep replenishment for our mind and body. We enter a theta brain state which allows us to rest deeply and rebalance. It can also often lead us into sleep as the body and mind relax and let go.

See Chapter 1, page 8, Chapter 4, page 55, and Chapter 8, page 109 for the yoga nidra scripts or listen to recordings via website.

Deliberate creating

Bring to mind things that you enjoy, for example, a feeling of security, spaciousness, fun, and contentment.

Allow yourself to feel the emotion connected to these states, bask in this vibration.

From here, you can make prayers and call forth that which you wish to increase in your life. It helps to keep it general, for example abundance, contentment, clarity (Hicks, 2004).

Herbal support

Soothing Chamomile tea before bedtime can help, as can using essential oils such as lavender and bergamot in a diffuser.

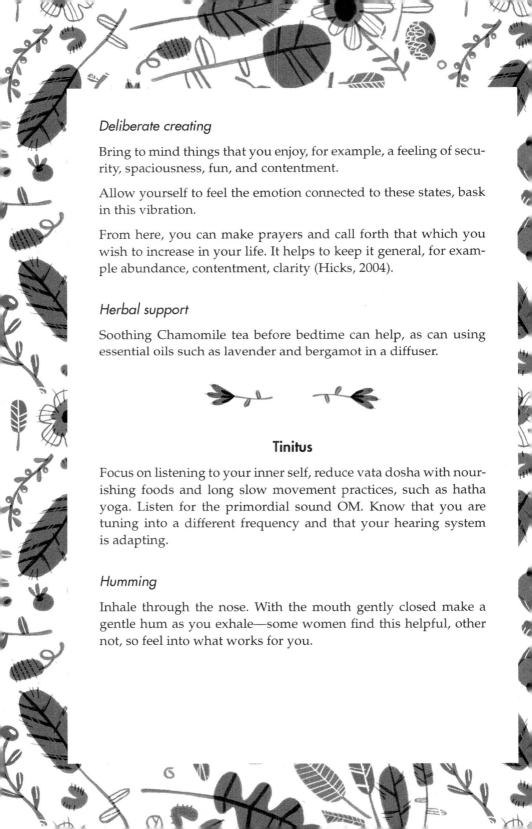

Tinitus

Focus on listening to your inner self, reduce vata dosha with nourishing foods and long slow movement practices, such as hatha yoga. Listen for the primordial sound OM. Know that you are tuning into a different frequency and that your hearing system is adapting.

Humming

Inhale through the nose. With the mouth gently closed make a gentle hum as you exhale—some women find this helpful, other not, so feel into what works for you.

Oiling the ear

An ancient ayurvedic practice of *sneehan*. Using a pipette put a few drops of warm sesame oil in each ear or ask a friend to do it for you. Relax and lie still for five minutes then drain the oil out of the ear. Do this regularly.

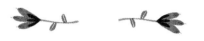

Vertigo

Much of our day is spent vertically. There may be a need to balance the vertical with the horizontal.

Stilling the body

Lie down and focus on your breath. Feel the earth supporting you.

Gentle movement

Make slow movements using the cross axis in the body. For example, lying on floor, lifting right leg and left arm then, left arm, right leg.

Experiment with simple balance poses, such as rooting down through one leg and then gently lifting the other behind you. Incorporating eye exercises[10] and head movements can also help.

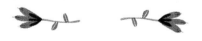

---

[10] Eye exercises may include bringing the gaze up towards the sky and back down, then to the ground, to the right, to the left. Repeat each position five times. At the end, rub the hands together to create heat and rest them on the eyes to relax (palming). This practice may not be suitable if you have cataracts or other eye conditions.

Hair Loss

Hair is linked to bones, our DNA, and ancestors. Hair loss is also related to unbalanced or increased vata dosha. Eating nourishing foods and reducing electronic use can help.

Massage scalp with oil

Use olive oil infused with rosemary, sesame oil or ayurvedic oil to stimulate the hair follicles and nourish the scalp.

Ancestral ritual

Our hair contains our DNA, that which holds our genetic information and functioning. Our DNA pattern relates to our ancestors, those that have walked before us. It may be that we hold challenging or unwanted aspects, including trauma, from our ancestors as well as the favourable qualities. By consciously engaging with our ancestral lineage and holding space for ritual and ceremony we can release and let go of certain aspects that we have inherited. The hair can be seen as linked to these patterns and by bringing more balance and releasing trauma it may be possible to enliven and nourish the hair.

See Chapter 3, page 42 for guidance.

Body massage

Warm a little sesame or olive oil by standing the cup of oil in a bowl of hot water. Take your time with this practice, being aware of the sensation and luxuriate in the self-care.

Apply the oil to the skin using long, slow, firm touch. Move from the middle body including hips, buttocks and waist and then move down the legs. At the joints, the knees, ankles and hips you can apply the oil in a circular motion.

Work along the sides of the body, around the navel (clockwise, once or twice), on the lower back. Reaching as much of the back as possible.

Circle the shoulders, elbows and wrists and move down the arms, applying oil to the hands and fingers. Continue by applying oil to the breasts in circular motions and armpits.

Apply the oil to the neck, shoulders and gently to the face. Use the fingertips to gently tap and then pinch along the eyebrows and jaw line. Oil can be applied to the scalp if you wish.

If possible, lie down on an old towel, making sure you are warm enough and rest, allowing the oil to absorb into the tissues of the body for 10–20 minutes. You can then have a warm shower, without using products.

(It is a good idea to pour a kettle of boiling water down the shower drain after you have finished your practice to prevent any issues with the drainage.)

In Ayurveda, the practice of oiling reduces vata dosha imbalance that is related to hair thinning and loss.

Use of ghee

Incorporating ghee into your diet can help as it reduces vata dosha, associated with hair loss. See Hale Pule in reference section, or another ayurvedic practitioner for more information about ghee and its uses.

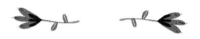

Dry skin

The skin is our boundary to the external world, a place of meetings, receiving, and letting go. Nourish this process and boundary.

Skin awareness

Be aware of the contact between your skin and the outside world as you go about your day. Notice how some sensations and experiences may be pleasing and others not.

Take time to breathe through the skin, allow yourself to ingest the nourishing light from the sun or moon through your body boundary.

Oiling the skin

The practice of oiling the skin not only allows us to give ourselves care and love but the long strokes on the skin relax our nervous system. Ideally leave the oil on for twenty minutes at least to allow it to soak into the deeper layers of the skin, replenishing the elasticity.

Warm a little sesame or olive oil by standing the cup of oil in a bowl of hot water. Take your time with this practice, being aware of the sensation and luxuriate in the self-care.

Apply the oil to the skin using long, slow, firm touch. Move from the middle body including hips, buttocks and waist and then move down the legs. At the joints, the knees, ankles and hips you can apply the oil in a circular motion.

Work along the sides of the body, around the navel (clockwise, once or twice), on the lower back. Reaching as much of the back as possible.

Circle the shoulders, elbows and wrists and move down the arms, applying oil to the hands and fingers. Continue by applying oil to the breasts in circular motions and armpits.

Apply the oil to the neck, shoulders and gently to the face. Use the fingertips to gently tap and then pinch along the eyebrows and jaw line. Oil can be applied to the scalp if you wish.

If possible, lie down on an old towel, making sure you are warm enough and rest, allowing the oil to absorb into the tissues of the body. You can then have a warm shower, without using products.

(It is a good idea to pour a kettle of boiling water down the shower drain after you have finished your practice to prevent any issues with the drainage.)

Internal oiling

Incorporating ghee into your diet can help. Ghee can reduce vata dosha imbalance which is associated with hair loss. See Hale Pule in reference section, or another ayurvedic practitioner for more information about ghee and its uses.

A space for your own insights, experiences, and images

_____

_____

_____

_____

_____

_____

_____

_____

_____

_____

_____

_____

_____

_____

_____

_____

CONCLUSION

As we challenge conditioned perceptions and perspectives around the menopause, we create a space for new exploration, and a new paradigm of thoughts and feelings. Through using the framework of initiation and rite of passage, we support ourselves in experiencing the menopause within a context of hope and new beginnings. As we are dismembered in the fire of yoga or the alchemical crucible during the climax of our menopausal process, we can hold somewhere in our consciousness or awareness that through this journey we will emerge with new skills, gifts, clarity, and awareness. There can be a thread of hope and trust that weaves alongside the rage and grief of our dismemberment. There will be jewels and gold to unearth and mine.

As with all initiations we experience a separation and severance from what and who we were, we face symbolic death and whilst in the underworld we experience intense emotions including fear, rage, grief, and the futility of life. We are taken apart and then re-woven. We then begin to emerge, assimilate and reintegrate, joining our community once more in a new way, with new understanding and knowledge.

Through conscious menopause we search for a meaningful connection with our whole self, all of our personality and our soul. Through the integration of our unconscious or hidden, shadow aspects we can move into a new phase of maturation.

As Simon Haas says in his exploration of the Bhagavad Gita, as a text to guide us through our own dark night;

> "Fear, lamentation and confusion disappear, leading to one's good fortune. A strong impulse to retreat from life gives way to unusual triumph, complete helplessness is replaced by strength and the revealing of our dark side leads to abiding wise conduct." (Haas, 2018)

During our journey we inhabit the in-between places, the non-linear, liminal, ethereal space. We drop into the underworld to face our fears, traumas, and pain. As our ovaries let go of our fertile eggs, we may look into the mirror and not recognise ourselves anymore, the roles we held dear seem foreign, and resonate with us no more. We put them down, not knowing if there is anything to replace them. We face our resistance to the conditioned view of the old hag, crone, and witch. Paradoxically, we know that she is what we seek and who will guide us into a new paradigm and rebirth.

With this awareness and knowing that our consciousness or psyche is undergoing a profound change we can accept and tolerate our experiences or symptoms with greater ease. When we perceive everything as energy and vibration, we can understand that our bodies and conscious mind will take time to adjust and integrate the unconscious and the energy changes that we are going through. As we assimilate these subtle energetic shifts, our minds and bodies adjust on cellular and energetic levels, we experience the growing pains and eventually move into the rubedo phase or the new state that has been arrived at.

In terms of my own process, I would say that my 'gold' is still being cleaned and refined, I feel that I am not yet fully 'through' my menopause journey. At the time of writing, I have not bled for over two years—this book is part of my process and part of the initiate's gift. It was a seed that I was not even aware that I had planted, and it has come to fruit as I near the end of my menopause passage.

Depending on where you are on your journey you may be feeling seeds taking form, perhaps they are still formless, or perhaps they are bearing fruit. Some of the gold from your initiatory process may be that your wounds are integrated in a different way, that certain qualities or traits are emphasised, or you now feel more able to give them freer expression.

I can see that part of the gifts I have harvested are that of discernment, particularly in terms of what I do with my time and who I do it with. I also have clarity that I am the wise woman that I was seeking. I know that my greatest teacher, lover, and friend is within. This knowing has allowed me to expand my confidence, to feel more anchored and have the capacity to follow my own energy and my own song, with less concern about what others think. I can rest more fully in trusting the greater mystery and universal tapestry. Part of that never-ending creative expansion includes my deliberate creation and that I have choices about what I create within that. We all have a unique passage and follow our own breadcrumb trail.

The menopause journey or 'the change' of life teaches us about change. That identity, role, and the people and places in our lives are mutable. Like the wind, they shift and transform as we do. Our changes in our internal landscape create the changes in our external reality. The process of metamorphosis is painful, uncomfortable, and uncertain, yet to resist and not change brings dis-eases, stagnation, and resentment. When we consciously engage with our spiritual path to keep growing, we draw upon the courage of the warrior and can be surprised that there is peace after the battle. As the heron reminded me, the spiritual warrior also requires patience. There is a divine order to things that at times can be obscured from our view.

Our bodies know that when we reconnect with them as a subtle, complex instrument we have the feedback we need about the steps we take. Similarly, our emotional guidance system is always there, are we moving towards our joy or away from it? When we are in the throes of menopause, we can doubt the initiatory journey that we are on. When I felt this, I cried to Grandmother and she reassured me 'do not fret, you are in the loom'. Our practice is to keep listening to our soul nudges and trust that all is unfolding perfectly. We are being weaved as we collect our new threads and learn to spin and weave once again. The journey to the underworld and immersion in the crucible is a profound catalyst for spiritual growth.

We learn from whom and what we can, and we find the nourishment and comfort that we need from the allies on our journey. As explored in this book, the cycles of nature and the elements always bring deep sustenance.

When we have journeyed through menopause, we have grieved for our physical womb and eggs. We hold the knowing of a different fertility; we know that our womb cauldron holds wisdom for the next generations. Our bodies changed, embody the journey that we have been on, a coat woven from both the wounds and pleasures. We step further into our maturation or individuation.

We are finding a new way, our mothers and grandmothers did not navigate menopause in the way we are feeling called to do, we have not had the role models. We may not feel ready or prepared for this journey, but like it or not, we are the way-showers for the women that follow. We navigate the best we can, knowing that the women who follow will hopefully benefit from our efforts and will surely expand and develop the trail from where we have left it.

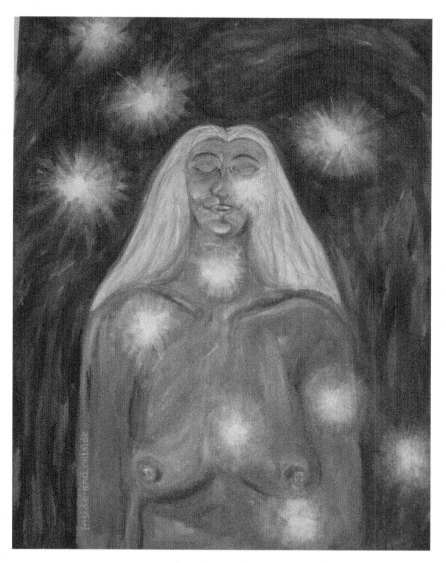

Wise Woman Interior Stars

APPENDIX 1

Chakras

Specific parts of the body are reference or focal points for subtle energy wheels. In many spiritual traditions these centres are recognised, and different practices are used to energise and balance them. Some of the different names used for them include transformative keys, interior stars, and dragon jewels. The chakras can deepen our self-understanding and as we refine and awaken these energy wheels, they support our inner awakening.

There are the primary six spinal chakras or energy wheels, although there are many more throughout the body. They primary chakras are along the central energy channel or nadi called sushumna nadi. Here I give a brief overview, but I would recommend a deeper exploration of the chakras through reading and practices. The simplest practice being awareness and breath at each focal point in the body associated with each chakra.

In yoga and tantra each chakra is associated with specific symbols and *bija or* seed mantra. These can vary between different traditions. The initial three chakras are mainly associated with our egoic perspective and self-orientation. The chakras that follow, open us to a greater awareness of our place within the bigger cosmic picture and support us in refining ourselves to being spirituality embodied. *Sahasrara*, located at the crown of the head is transcendence, and beyond the concept of duality. I refer to the chakras at different times in the book.

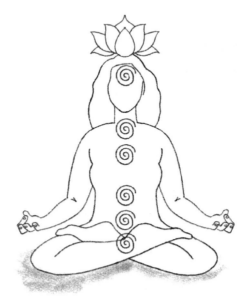

Chakras

Mooladhara or root chakra

Moola is root, *adhara* is foundation.

Located for women inside the vagina, between the vaginal opening and the cervix.

It is linked to our foundations and the earth, hence 'root'. It is connected to our primitive survival needs, that of shelter, food, warmth, and procreation. This foundation is often severely shaken during menopause, as discussed in Chapter 1, 'Red River Runs Dry'.

Symbols include an earthy red colour and an elephant.

The bija mantra is LAM (pronounced *LUM*).

Swadisthana chakra

Swa one's own, *adhisthana* is abode.

Located in the pelvic or sacral area, in front of the coccyx and behind the pubic bone.

Concerned with sexuality and sensuality. Pleasure via the senses and personal gratification. Associated with the unconscious and instinctual drives. Often given a negative press, but it actually can support us in reconnecting with our creativity, embodied divine love and sacred sexuality as discussed in Chapter 7, 'The Priestess is in the Temple'.

Symbols include the colour orange, deep water, a half-alligator half-dolphin animal and the crescent moon.

Bija mantra is VAM (pronounced *VUM*).

Manipura chakra

Mani is jewel, *pura* is city.

The city of jewels is located at the navel, behind the belly button.

It is the centre of personal will, energy, our power and dynamic expression in the world. It is linked with strong emotions such as anger, rage, impotence, and anxiety that we meet during menopause. It is what we harness as we move into our crone-dom and sovereignty to have the confidence to take our gifts into the world.

Symbols include our inner sun, the colour yellow, a ram.

Bija mantra is RAM (pronounced *RUM*).

Anahata chakra

Anahata means unstruck or sound without vibration.

Located in the centre of the chest.

The heart space is seen as our centre, our connection with expanded perception beyond ego. Linked to finer qualities and attributes of compassion, love, empathy, and trust in life. As we move into our sovereignty and wise woman, we sit in the heart space.

Symbols include a light green, pink or blue colour, the deer or antelope, and a six-pointed star.

Bija mantra is YAM (pronounced *YUM*).

Vishuddhi chakra

Vishuddhi means purification.

Located at the centre of the throat.

Associated with communication, expression, discrimination and purification.

Vishuddhi is the seat of communication, speaking our truth, being clear and expressing our sound in the world, which can include singing and chanting. This is an important chakra during menopause as it aligns us with our authenticity, clarity and truth speaking and letting go of old ways of communicating.

Symbols include the swan of discernment, a sky-blue colour, and a drop of nectar.

Bija mantra is HAM (pronounced *HUM*).

Agya chakra

Agya means command, also known as the third eye.

Located at the centre of the head, the focal point being at the eyebrow centre.

This is the seat of wisdom, intuition, clarity, the *seer*.

Symbols include an eagle soaring in a vast sky, the colour indigo, the sun and moon representing duality.

Bija mantra is OM (pronounced *AUM*).

Beyond these six primary chakras is the sahasrara:

Sahasrara

Meaning *thousand* or infinite.

Located at the crown of the head.

Represented by a thousand petal lotus flower.

This is beyond the conscious mind and awareness. Here the individual meets the transcendental and cosmic. Here duality is integrated. This is the seat of the fulfilment of spiritual awakening, fullness in the emptiness.

INDEX OF PRACTICES

Some of these practices are available as a free audio recording at the School of the Sacred Feminine website (schoolofthesacredfeminine. co.uk)

Chapter 1

Chapter 2

Chapter 3

Chapter 4

Chapter 5

Chapter 6

Chapter 7

Chapter 8

REFERENCES

Introduction

1. Jones, Rosalyn, *https://henpicked.net* (last accessed 16/05/22)
2. Jones, Rosalyn, *https://henpicked.net* (last accessed 16/05/22)
3. Odier, Daniel, *Tantric Kali* (Vermont, Inner Traditions, 2016) page 3
4. Kindred, Glennie, *The Earth's Cycle of Celebration* (Glennie Kindred Publication, 1991)
5. Selbie, Joseph, Steinmetz, David, *The Yugas: Keys to Understanding Our Hidden Past, Emerging Energy Age and Enlightened Future* (Crystal Clarity Publications, 2011) page 96

Chapter 1

1. Pope, Alexanadra, *https://www.redschool.net* (last accessed 12/02/2022)
2. Odier, Daniel, *Desire, The Tantric Path to Awakening* (Vermont, Inner Traditions, 1999) page 89
3. Amélie, Noack, *The Matrix as Container and Crucible* (IGA Learning Experience April, 2017) page 4
4. Mankowitz, Ann, *Change of Life* (Inner City Books, 1984) page 57
5. Mankowitz, Ann, *Change of Life* (Inner City Books, 1984) page 66

Chapter 2

1. Odier, Danial, *Desire, The Tantric Path to Awakening* (Vermont, Inner Traditions, 1999) page 94
2. Blackie, Sharon, *The Chronicles of Old Crane Woman*
3. Gifford, Jo, *https://www.outdoorswimmingsociety.com* (last accessed 18/07/2022)
4. Odier, Daniel, *Tantric Kali* (Vermont, Inner Traditions, 2016) page 12
5. Roth, Gabrielle, *5 Rhythms* www.5rhythms.com (last accessed 15/06/22)
6. Buxton, Simon, *The Shamanic Way of the Bee* (Vermont, Destiny Books, 2004) page 114

Chapter 3

1. Haas, Simon, *Yoga and the Dark night of the Soul* (London, Veda Wisdom Books, 2018) page 79
2. Rosenherg, Stanley, *Accessing the Healing Power of the Vagus Nerve* (North Atlantic books, 2017)
3. Odier, Daniel, *Tantric Kali* (Vermont, Inner Traditions, 2016) page 9
4. https://thyroiduk.org/ (last accessed 26/10/2022)
5. Buxton, Simon, *The Shamanic Way of the Bee* (Vermont, Destiny Books, 2004) page 114

Chapter 4

1. Emoto, Masuru, *The Hidden Messages in Water* (Atria Books, 2005) page 94
2. Satyasanananda, Swami, *Tattwa Shuddhi* (Bihar, Yoga Publications, 1984) page 64

Chapter 5

1. Reinhart, Melanie, *Chiron and the Healing Journey* (Starwalker Press, London, 1989) page 293
2. Reinhart, Melanie, *Chiron and the Healing Journey* (Starwalker Press, London, 1989) page 25
3. Reinhart, Melanie, *Chiron and the Healing Journey* (Starwalker Press, London, 1989) page 63

4. Blackie, Sharon, *If Women Rose Rooted* (UK, September Publications, 2019) page 123

5. Brofman, Martin, *Anything can be healed* (Vermont, Findhorn Press, 2003) page 27

6. Reinhart M, *Chiron and the Healing Journey* (Starwalker Press, London, 1989) page 292

7. Rosenherg, Stanley, *Accessing the Healing Power of the Vagus Nerve* (North Atlantic books 2017) page 11

8. Buxton, Simon, *The Shamanic Way of the Bee* (Vermont, Destiny Books, 2004) page 48

Chapter 7

1. Sharman-Burke, Greene Liz, *The Mythic Tarot* (Rider, 1995) page 30

2. Deida, David, *The Way of the Superior Man* (Sounds True, 2017) page 52

3. Buxton, Simon, *The Shamanic Way of the Bee* (Vermont, Destiny Books, 2004) page 110

4. Minke de vos Minke des Vos, *Tao Tantric Arts for Women* (Canada, Destiny Books, 2016) page 210

5. Long, Barry, *Making Love, Sexual Love the Divine Way* (London, Barry Long Books, 1998) page 37

6. Anand, Margo, *The Art of Sexual Ecstasy* (UK, Jeremey P Tarcher, 1991) page 144

7. Minke des Vos, *Tao Tantric Arts for Women* (Canada, Destiny Books, 2016) p181

8. Long, Barry, *Making Love, Sexual Love the Divine Way* (London, Barry Long Books, 1998) page 27

9. Buxton, Simon, *The Shamanic Way of the Bee* (Vermont, Destiny Books, 2004) p 114

10. Kenyan Tom, Sion J, *The Magdalen Manuscript* (ORB Communications, 2002) page 49

11. Long, Barry, *Making Love, Sexual Love the Divine Way* (London, Barry Long Books, 1998) page 5

12. Deida, David, *The Enlightened Sex Manual* (Colorado, Sounds True, 2004) page 4

13. Anand, Margo, *The Art of Sexual Ecstasy* (UK, Jeremey P Tarcher, 1991) page 96

14. Swami Satyananda, Saraswati, *Asana Pranayama Mudra Bandha* (Bihar, Yoga Publications Trust 1969) page 385

Chapter 8

1. Rodrigues Maria, Lippert Trenton, Nguyen Hung, *Menstrual Blood-Derived Stem Cells: In Vitro and In Vivo Characterization of Functional Effects* (2016) (last accessed 15/10/22)
2. Sharman-Burke, Greene Liz, *The Mythic Tarot* (Rider, 1995) page 55
3. Sharman-Burke, Greene Liz, *The Mythic Tarot* (Rider, 1995) page 55
4. *Spider woman* as found in the Native American Navaho tradition- (compiled by Ann Dunbar handout, 2007)
5. Bake Tom van, *Hiranyagarbha ('Golden Egg') and Prajapati ('Creation Lord') on Indus seals* (2018)
6. Ursula Le Guin cited by Mankowitz, Ann, *Change of Life* (Inner City Books, 1984) page 109
7. Hicks, Esther and Jerry, *Ask and it is Given* (London, Hay House, 2004) page 53
8. Banafsheh Sayyad, *Sacred Sufi Dance, Cultivate Body of Light* (course via Shift Network, 2022, last accessed 27/06/2022)

Chapter 10

1. www.menopausematters.co.uk (last accessed 26/10/2022)

Conclusion

1. Haas, Simon, *Yoga and the Dark night of the Soul* (London, Veda Wisdom Books, 2018) page 114

BIBLIOGRAPHY

Anand, Margo, *The Art of Sexual Ecstasy* (UK, Jeremey P Tarcher, 1991)

Blackie, Sharon, *If Women Rose Rooted* (UK, September Publications, 2019)

Buxton, Simon, *The Shamanic Way of the Bee* (Vermont, Destiny Books, 2004)

Brofman, Martin, *Anything can be healed* (Vermont, Findhorn Press, 2003)

Darrell, Nikki, *Conversation with Plants* (Aeon Books, 2020)

Deida, David, *The Enlightened Sex Manual* (Colorado, Sounds True, 2004)

Deida, David, *The Way of the Superior Man* (Sounds True, 2017)

Dinsmore-Tulsi, Uma, *Yoni Shakti* (Yoga Words, 2014)

Egoscue, Pete, *www.egoscue.com* (last accessed 22/05/2022)

Haas, Simon, *Yoga and the Dark night of the Soul* (London, Veda Wisdom Books, 2018)

Hicks, Esther and Jerry, *Ask and it is Given* (London, Hay House, 2004)

Kempton, Sally, *Awakening Shakti* (Colorado, Sounds True, 2013)

Kenyan Tom, Sion J, *The Magdalen Manuscript* (ORB Communications, 2002)

Kindred Glennie, *The Earth's Cycle of Celebration* (Glennie Kindred Publication, 1991)

Lewin, Myra, *Freedom in your Relationship with Food* (Myra Lewin Publication, 2017)

Long, Barry, *Making Love, Sexual Love the Divine Way* (London, Barry Long Books, 1998)

Mankowitz, Ann, *Change of Life* (Inner City Books, 1984)

Minke des Vos, *Tao Tantric Arts for Women* (Canada, Destiny Books, 2016)

Noack, Amélie, *The Matrix as Container and Crucible* (IGA Learning experience paper, 2017)

Odier, Danial, *Desire, The Tantric Path to Awakening* (Vermont, Inner Traditions, 1999)

Odier, Daniel, *Tantric Kali* (Vermont, Inner Traditions, 2016)

Pinkola Estes C, *Women who run with Wolves* (Rider, 2008)

Pixie, Magenta, *The Infinite Helix and the Emerald Flame* (White Spirit Publishing, 2018)

Plotkin, Bill, *Soul Craft* (New World Library, 2003)

Pope, Alexandra, *Wild Power* (UK, Hayhouse, 2017)

Reinhart M, *Chiron and the Healing Journey* (Starwalker Press, London, 1989)

Rosenberg, Stanley, *Accessing the Healing Power of the Vagus Nerve* (North Atlantic Books, US, 2017)

Satyasanananda, Swami, *Tattwa Shuddhi* (Bihar, Yoga Publications, 1984)

Weed, Susan, *New Menopausal Years, the Wise Woman Way* (Ash Tree Publishing, NY, 2002)

Selbie, Joseph, Steinmetz, David, *The Yugas: Keys to Understanding Our Hidden Past, Emerging Energy Age and Enlightened Future* (Crystal Clarity Publications, 2011)

Sharman-Burke, Greene Liz, *The Mythic Tarot* (Rider, 1995)

Swami Satyananda, Saraswati, *Asana Pranayama Mudra Bandha* (Bihar, Yoga Publications Trust 1969)

FURTHER RESOURCES

Founded by author Revā Adie offering inspiration, events and practices to support women and men on their human, sacred journey
www.schoolofthesacredfeminine.co.uk
Red School—Menopause Podcasts *www.redschool.net*
Yoga Nidra website—recordings of Yoga Nidra available for download
www.yoganidranetwork.org/downloads
Agnihotra—Information and guidance to hold daily sacred fires *www.
agnihotra.org*
Mandala Yoga Ashram—Yoga and Tantra courses, retreats, and blog *www.
mandalayogaashram.com*
The Sacred Trust—Shamanic courses, including courses in Lyceum
sacredtrust.org
Hale Pule—Ayurveda courses, podcasts, how to make ghee, and blog
www.halepule.com
The Herb Society—information about herbs *herbsociety.org.uk*
National Institute of Medical Herbalists *nimh.org.uk*
Menopause Matters—information primarily from medical perspective
www.menopausematters.co.uk
Thyroid UK—information about thyroid imbalance including alternatives
to synthetic medication and community support *thyroiduk.org*

ACKNOWLEDGEMENTS

Many thanks to all those that have supported me, not only in the writing of this book but on my journey. That includes all my teachers, foremost Siddha Yoga, those at The Sacred Trust and Mandala Yoga Ashram, especially my dear friend Swami Krishnapremananda. To my birth family, especially my mother for her guidance, love and understanding. To my sister for her support and proofreading. To 'the valley' and Emerald for sharing the beauty, magic, and wildness of unspoilt land. To all the women who have shared authentically and courageously. Thanks to my dear friend Ron Warmington (IG: @warmron), for his patience and artwork. To dancing Jo Brown for reading the draft, helpful suggestions and for sweet encouragement from Divyagopi, and to my Turvey friends for accepting and believing in me.

ABOUT THE AUTHOR

Through her writing and teaching Revā weaves together her extensive spiritual experience and knowledge. She has been exploring the deeper mysteries of life and esoteric aspects of spirituality for over thirty years. Her writing conveys her understanding of the human predicament and our need to embrace the re-awakening of the Divine feminine. She is passionate about supporting women and men on their spiritual and healing journeys, encouraging balance through connection with nature and Source, moving us nearer to authenticity, joy and freedom.

schoolofthesacredfeminine.co.uk

INDEX